Medicinal Chemistry

Medicinal Chemistry

A Look at How Drugs Are Discovered

A. K. Ganguly and Sesha Sridevi Alluri

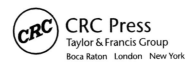

CRC Press
Taylor & Francis Group
Boca Raton London New York

CRC Press is an imprint of the
Taylor & Francis Group, an **informa** business

First edition published 2022
by CRC Press
6000 Broken Sound Parkway NW, Suite 300
Boca Raton, FL 33487–2742

and by CRC Press
2 Park Square, Milton Park, Abingdon, Oxon, OX14 4RN

© 2022 A. K. Ganguly, Sesha Sridevi Alluri

CRC Press is an imprint of Taylor & Francis Group, LLC

Library of Congress Cataloging-in-Publication Data

Names: Ganguly, A. K., author. | Alluri, Sesha Sridevi, author.
Title: Medicinal chemistry : a look at how drugs are discovered / A.K.
    Ganguly, Sesha Sridevi Alluri.
Description: First edition. | Boca Raton : Taylor and Francis, 2022. |
    Includes bibliographical references and index.
Identifiers: LCCN 2021023343 (print) | LCCN 2021023344 (ebook) | ISBN
    9781032017532 (paperback) | ISBN 9781032022536 (hardback) | ISBN
    9781003182573 (ebook)
Subjects: LCSH: Pharmaceutical chemistry. | Chemotherapy.
Classification: LCC RS403 .G36 2022 (print) | LCC RS403 (ebook) | DDC
    615.1/9—dc23
LC record available at https://lccn.loc.gov/2021023343
LC ebook record available at https://lccn.loc.gov/2021023344

ISBN: 978-1-032-02253-6 (hbk)
ISBN: 978-1-032-01753-2 (pbk)
ISBN: 978-1-003-18257-3 (ebk)

DOI: 10.1201/9781003182573

Typeset in Times
by Apex CoVantage, LLC

Contents

Preface

The discovery of drugs involves an interdisciplinary approach, particularly with regard to synthetic organic chemistry, without which, by definition, no new synthetic drugs can be discovered. Collaborations with biologists involved in various aspects, including those involved in animal experiments, and toxicologists are essential. Drug discovery is a very complex, time-consuming, and expensive process. However, the discovery of so many spectacular drugs for curing various diseases over a period of decades has demonstrated the ingenuity of the human mind, and as one looks into the future, it is not too risky to speculate that newer medicines will be discovered for existing diseases and those yet to be encountered.

The discovery of penicillin during the Second World War not only saved many lives but was also the serious beginning of modern-day drug discovery. Penicillin was discovered by fermentation of a microorganism isolated from natural sources, as were the vast majority of anti-infectives, such as erythromycin, vancomycin, and tetracyclines, used in human medicine. Plants have also been rich sources of drugs, including Taxol, vincristine, and reserpine. It should also be noted that the origins of several other drugs can be traced back to compounds obtained from natural sources. For example, 6-aminopenicillanic acid is the starting material for the preparation of the well-known beta-lactam antibiotics. Similarly, Taxotere, a potent anticancer agent, is derived from the natural product 10-deacetylbaccatin III. Lovastatin, a cholesterol-lowering agent, is likewise derived from a natural product. In all these instances synthetic organic chemists made very important contributions. Research in steroids in the 1950s attracted many brilliant chemists of the day, as evidenced by the number of Nobel Prizes awarded in this area of research. Once again, the starting point for manufacturing all the steroids was the plant-derived diosgenin. It provided a cheap starting material with the required rigid ring structure and absolute stereo-chemistry of steroids. However, the majority of drugs discovered since the 1980s have been small molecules, thanks to major advancements made in various areas of biology, computational chemistry, and x-ray crystallography of proteins as well as continuing advances in synthetic organic chemistry. As many drugs are chiral, special attention has been paid to developing efficient chiral synthesis.

In the present book we have tried to capture all these areas, albeit not exhaustively. Our intention, at the end of the day, was to make medicinal chemistry an exciting and rewarding area of study. After all, what could be more satisfying than discovering a drug that can cure serious diseases and possibly save some lives?

ACKNOWLEDGMENTS

We wish to thank Dr. N. Y. Shih, former Senior Director of Research at Schering-Plough Research Institute, for reading the entire manuscript and making helpful suggestions.

Authors

A.K. Ganguly, PhD, was born in India and educated in India and England. He attended the Imperial College of Science and Technology, London, where he earned his PhD in chemistry in 1961 under the supervision of Sir Derek Barton, a Nobel Laureate in chemistry. After finishing his studies at the Imperial College, Prof. Ganguly returned to India to work for Glaxo Laboratories and, later, with the Ciba Research Center in Bombay. He immigrated to the USA in 1967, and after a brief stay at the Research Institute of Medicine and Chemistry, Cambridge, Massachusetts, he joined Schering-Plough Research Institute, Kenilworth, New Jersey, in 1968 as a senior scientist and advanced to the position of Senior Vice President of Chemical Research. He is associated with the discovery of Zetia, posaconazole, lonafarnib, and boceprevir. Prof. Ganguly is a coauthor of 222 papers and coinventor with joint ownership of 88 patents. He has received several awards, including the E.B. Hershberg Award for Important Discoveries in Medicinally Active Substances from the American Chemical Society. After retiring from Schering-Plough, he joined Stevens Institute of Technology, Hoboken, New Jersey, as a distinguished research professor of chemistry and presently continues to consult in the drug discovery area.

Sesha Sridevi Alluri, PhD, earned her MSc degree in medicinal chemistry in India, and after working as a senior chemist at Dr. Reddy's Laboratories for a few years, she immigrated to the United States and joined Stevens Institute of Technology, Hoboken, New Jersey. She earned a second MS degree and PhD from the institute under the supervision of Prof. A.K. Ganguly. Presently, Prof. Alluri is working as a lecturer in the Department of Chemistry and Chemical Biology at Stevens Institute. She teaches undergraduate and graduate chemistry courses, including medicinal chemistry, and supervises undergraduate students in organic synthesis research projects. She is the recipient of several awards, including the ACS/WCC/Eli Lilly Award.

1 Introduction to Drug Discovery

1.1 DRUG DISCOVERY

Drug discovery[1–3] is a complex process and begins with the selection of a biochemical target of the disease, which involves a specific enzyme or receptor, and the assays are assembled by biologists for screening purposes. With high-throughput screening in place, chemical compounds obtained from collections—usually in the millions—in the files of pharmaceutical industries are tested; this is generally the case, particularly in the discovery of receptor agonists/antagonists. This is because structural information of receptors is not usually available. However, in the case of discovery of enzyme inhibitors, several different approaches are possible in addition to the screening of available compounds in the files. Unlike receptors, the structures of several enzymes have been determined using x-ray crystallography. It is particularly useful for optimization of an initial lead if the x-ray structure of the ligand bound to the enzyme is available. Once a lead structure has been identified, its selectivity against a panel of enzymes/receptors is determined. With a potent and selective compound in hand, it undergoes pharmacokinetic studies in several species of animals—usually rodents, dogs, and monkeys. The purpose of this study is to determine whether the active compound can be delivered orally, which is usually the preferred route of administration in humans, although drugs administered by intravenous or intramuscular routes are well known, and to determine how well it is **A**bsorbed, **D**istributed, **M**etabolized and **E**xcreted. Thus, these are usually referred to as ADME studies. The preferred compound with desired potency, selectivity, and pharmacokinetic properties is progressed to in vivo studies in a disease model, followed by three months of toxicity studies in rats and dogs. If the lead compound is found to have acceptable toxicity, the results are disclosed to the Food and Drug Administration (FDA) to obtain permission to investigate the drug candidate in the clinic; this is otherwise known as an IND (Investigational New Drug) application. The clinical trials are carried out in three phases. In phase 1 the drug is administered to healthy volunteers to determine a safe dose, then researchers proceed to phase 2 to determine efficacy in sick patients and, finally, to phase 3 to apply the drug to a broader patient population or compare it with an existing drug for the same disease. At each step the FDA has the opportunity to review the data, and before the drug is finally approved for human use, a toxicity study in animals lasting six months or longer is conducted. The whole process is lengthy, involves scientists of different disciplines, and is very expensive.

DOI: 10.1201/9781003182573-1

1.1.1 COMPOUND SCREENING AT PHARMACEUTICAL INDUSTRIES

Most drugs are derived by chemical synthesis or obtained from natural sources, and proteins are obtained by recombinant biotechnology. A few examples from each of the categories are cited in the following list.

1. Medicinal chemistry involving chemical synthesis: Claritin,[4] Zocor,[5] Lipitor,[6] Zetia,[7] captopril,[8] enalapril,[8] Zantac,[9] Valium,[10] Prozac,[11] Celebrex,[12] Januvia,[13] posaconazole,[14] ibuprofen,[15] Tylenol,[16] fluconazole,[17] linezolid.[18]
2. Drugs from natural sources or derived from compounds obtained from natural sources:
   Plants and microbes are sources of approximately half of the medicines used today. Some of the examples of drugs obtained from plants include *Vinca* alkaloids, reserpine, aspirin, and Taxol.[19] Major anti-infectives used in the clinic today are either produced by microorganisms obtained from soil samples or derived from compounds obtained from natural sources. These include penicillin, cephalosporins, aminoglycosides, erythromycin, amphotericin, and ivermectin. The discovery of Zocor, the first example of a cholesterol-lowering agent, can be traced back to natural sources. Steroids are produced by chemical modification of diosgenin, which is obtained from plants.
3. Biotechnology-derived drugs include introns, interleukins, Remicade, insulin,[20] human growth factors and several monoclonal antibodies. Immunotherapy is, of course, the most exciting development in human medicine today. However, a detailed discussion of this aspect of drug discovery is outside the scope of this book.
4. Structure-based drug discovery is an exciting area of drug discovery that has led to the discovery of protease inhibitors used in the treatment of HIV[21] and HCV[22] infections as well as many other diseases.
5. Combinatorial chemistry[23] is used to produce libraries of large numbers of compounds that are then screened in a high-throughput mode. This approach is widely used in the pharmaceutical industry. Although random and discovery libraries have been successful in identifying lead compounds, lead optimization using synthesis of focused libraries has been more successful. As this topic has been the subject matter of several books, it will not be discussed in this presentation.

1.1.2 LIPINSKI'S RULE

For drugs to be orally active, it is recommended that one follow Lipinski's rule of five,[24] which states that compounds with the following characteristics will have a better chance of success as orally active drugs:

1. Molecular weight <500
2. Fewer than ten hydrogen bond acceptors
3. Fewer than five hydrogen bond donors
4. CLogP <5 (lipophilicity)

1.2 DNA TO PROTEIN

Before we start learning about drug discovery, which will involve enzymes and receptors, it is important to have an appreciation of the structure and function of a very fundamental chemical in all our lives: DNA.[25] DNA carries genetic information of all lives and is a very simple construct, using only four bases: adenine (A), guanine (G), cytosine (C), and thymine (T). It also involves a sugar residue, deoxyribose, and phosphate linkages. The two strands of DNA containing ATGC bases in proper sequence are held together in the form of a double helix wherein A and T in the complementary single strands along with G and C are held together via hydrogen bonding (Figures 1.1–1.3). Thus, the hydrophobic ATGC bases are held together away from water and the phosphate linkages are solvent-exposed. It is to be noted

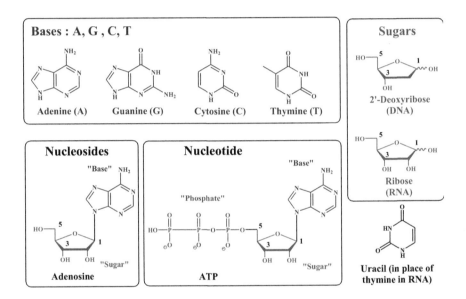

FIGURE 1.1   Structures of nucleic acid bases, sugars, nucleoside, nucleotide.

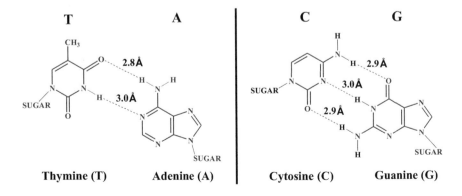

FIGURE 1.2   Hydrogen bonding between purine and pyrimidine bases.

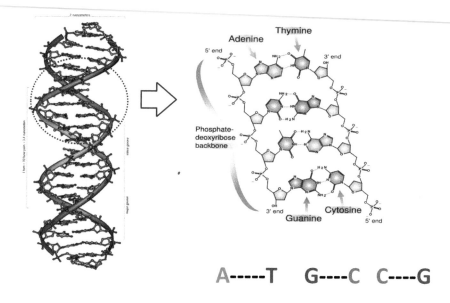

FIGURE 1.3 DNA double helix.

that adenine (A) and guanine (G) are purine bases, whereas cytosine (C) and thymine (T) are pyrimidines. In a double helical structure, two purine bases cannot pair via hydrogen bonding because they will be too close to each other; in the case of two pyrimidines, they cannot be complementary because they will be too far apart to form hydrogen bonding. However, a purine base is perfectly placed to form hydrogen bonding with a pyrimidine base in a complementary chain in the double helix.

The structures of A, G, C, and T are shown in Figure 1.1, as are those for adenosine, a nucleoside containing a 2-deoxyribose unit attached to adenine, and adenosine triphosphate (ATP), a nucleotide containing adenine attached to a 2-deoxyribose that in turn is phosphorylated. In the structure of RNA, the 2-deoxyribose moiety in DNA is replaced with ribose and thymine (T) is replaced with uracil (U).

Double helical DNA carries the genetic code of all living things, which is transcribed to single-stranded RNA, which in turn is translated to proteins (Figure 1.4). In the drug discovery process, one needs to be concerned with enzymes and receptors, both of which are proteins. Enzymes are smaller in size and often can be crystallized, and structures of several of them have been elucidated using x-ray crystallographic analysis. Receptors possess larger molecular weight, and as they are membrane-bound, it is very difficult to crystallize them.

The majority of drugs are either enzyme inhibitors, such as penicillin, which is a serine protease inhibitor, or receptor antagonists, such as Claritin, which is a histamine receptor antagonist; some are also receptor agonists. Once an initial lead is discovered, careful planning requires the optimization of the lead structure to a drug; for example, one should follow Lipinski's rule and avoid chemical groups that are known to be toxic (e.g., a Michael acceptor or alpha halo ketone). There has to always be a balance of activity and toxicity.

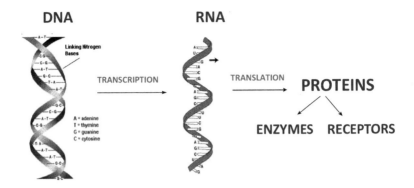

FIGURE 1.4 The central dogma of molecular biology.[26]

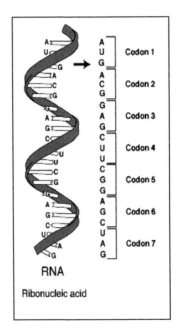

FIGURE 1.5 Triplet codons in mRNA.

Genes are linear sequences of nucleotides along a segment of DNA, which, when translated to RNA, carries a specific function. There are 20 naturally occurring amino acids, the structures of which are shown later, all of which, except glycine, possess an asymmetric center. Each amino acid is recognized in the RNA by specific triplet codes of nucleotides called codons. There are 64 codons, representing 20 amino acids, which means that some of the amino acids carry more than one specific triplet code and also incorporate stop codons (Figures 1.5 & 1.6).

Following are the structures of the 20 naturally occurring amino acids (Figure 1.7).

Second base in codon

	U	C	A	G	
U	UUU Phe UUC Phe UUA Leu UUG Leu	UCU Ser UCC Ser UCA Ser UCG Ser	UAU Tyr UAC Tyr UAA Stop UAG Stop	UGU Cys UGC Cys UGA Stop UGG Trp	U C A G
C	CUU Leu CUC Leu CUA Leu CUG Leu	CCU Pro CCC Pro CCA Pro CCG Pro	CAU His CAC His CAA Gln CAG Gln	CGU Arg CGC Arg CGA Arg CGG Arg	U C A G
A	AUU Ile´ AUC Ile AUA Ile AUG Met Start	ACU Thr ACC Thr ACA Thr ACG Thr	AAU Asn AAC Asn AAA Lys AAG Lys	AGU Ser AGC Ser AGA Arg AGG Arg	U C A G
G	GUU Val GUC Val GUA Val GUG Val	GCU Ala GCC Ala GCA Ala GCG Ala	GAU Asp GAC Asp GAA Glu GAG Glu	GGU Gly GGC Gly GGA Gly GGG Gly	U C A G

First base in codon (left vertical label) — Third base in codon (right vertical label)

FIGURE 1.6 Amino acids represented by 64 codons, including stop codons.

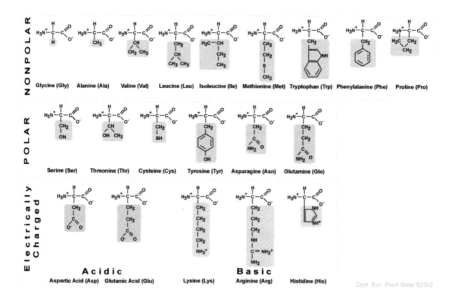

FIGURE 1.7 Structures of amino acids.

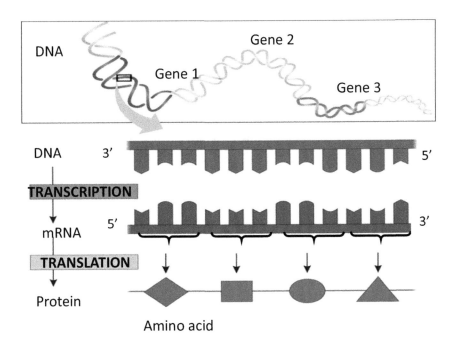

FIGURE 1.8 Transcription and translation to produce amino acid sequence.

DNA	... CGG CGA CCA ...
RNA	... GCC GCU GGU ...
AMINO ACID	... ALANINE—ALANINE—GLYCINE ...

FIGURE 1.9 Generation of hypothetical amino acid sequence from DNA.

In a hypothetical case the sequence CGG CGA CCA in a DNA strand will be transcribed in RNA as GCC GCU GGU, which in turn will be translated to ALANINE—ALANINE—GLYCINE. It should be noted that the triplet code for alanine could be GCC and GCU (Figures 1.8 & 1.9).

1.3 GROWING DNA CHAIN & REVERSE TRANSCRIPTASE INHIBITORS

During DNA replication, the 3' end, which has a hydroxyl (-OH) group on the deoxyribose sugar, covalently links to the phosphate at the 5' end of the incoming nucleotide to make phosphodiester bonds. The release of the two outer phosphate groups provides energy for the formation of the phosphodiester bond (Figure 1.10).

Reverse transcriptase (RT) inhibitors[27] are drugs used for the treatment of acquired immunodeficiency syndrome (AIDS) (Figure 1.11). Human immunodeficiency virus (HIV) is the causative agent of AIDS. A nucleoside analog, azidothymidine (AZT)[28]

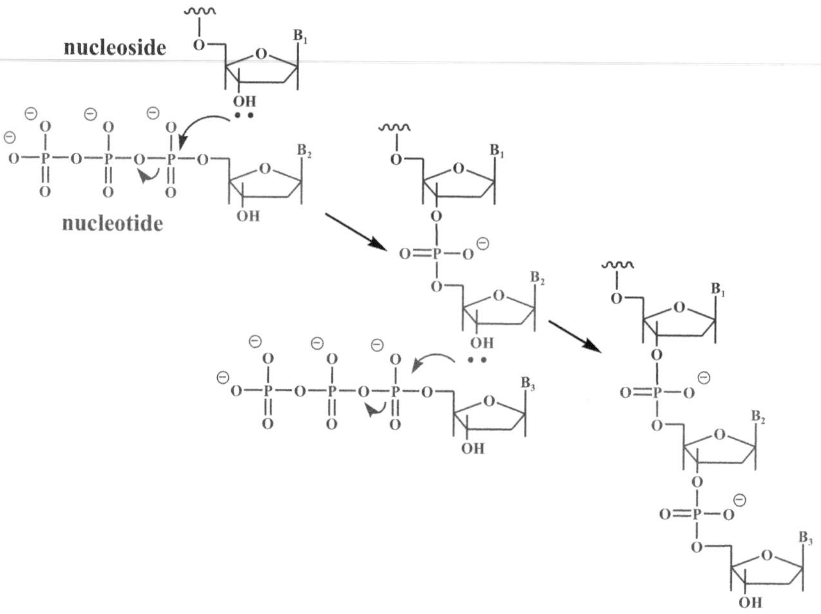

FIGURE 1.10 Growing DNA chain.

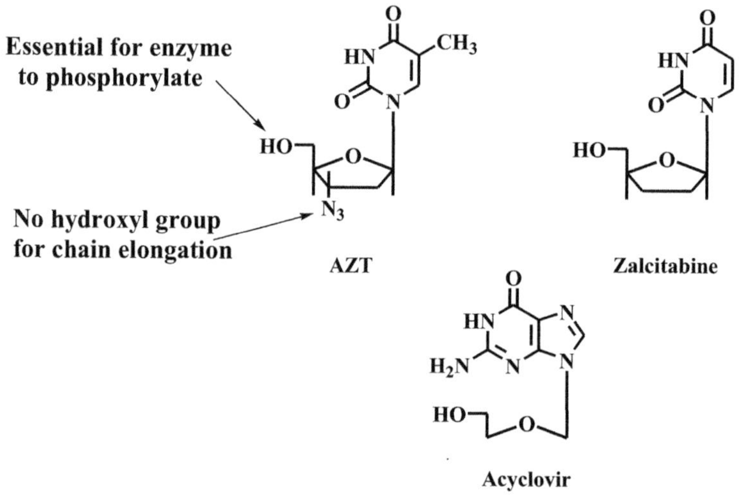

FIGURE 1.11 Examples of reverse transcriptase inhibitors.

works selectively by inhibiting HIV's RT, an enzyme the virus uses to make DNA from its RNA. AZT has a 3' hydroxyl group on the sugar moiety that has been replaced by an azido group. The kinase enzymes phosphorylate AZT to its active 5-triphosphate metabolite. AZT then gets incorporated into the growing DNA chain of the virus following steps similar to those illustrated in Figure 1.10, resulting in chain termination (Figure 1.12).

The synthesis of AZT from thymidine is shown in Scheme 1.1.

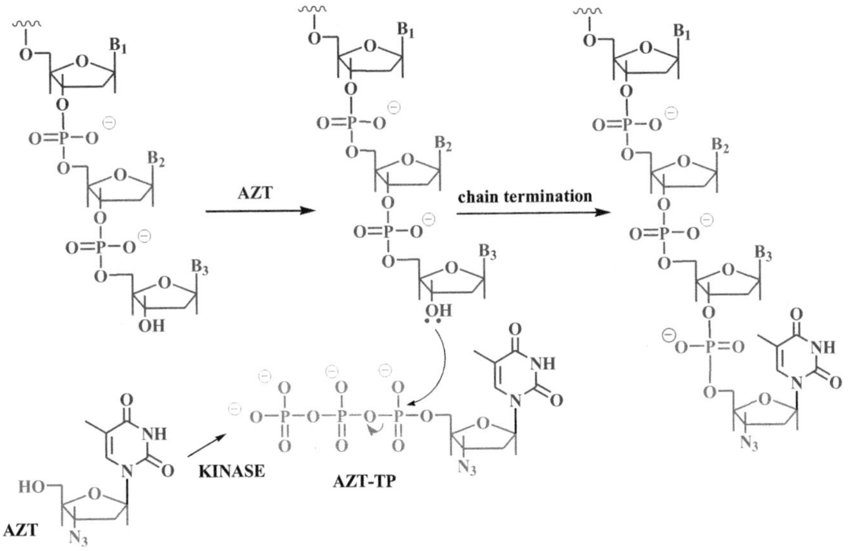

FIGURE 1.12 Incorporation of AZT into the growing DNA chain of the HIV virus.

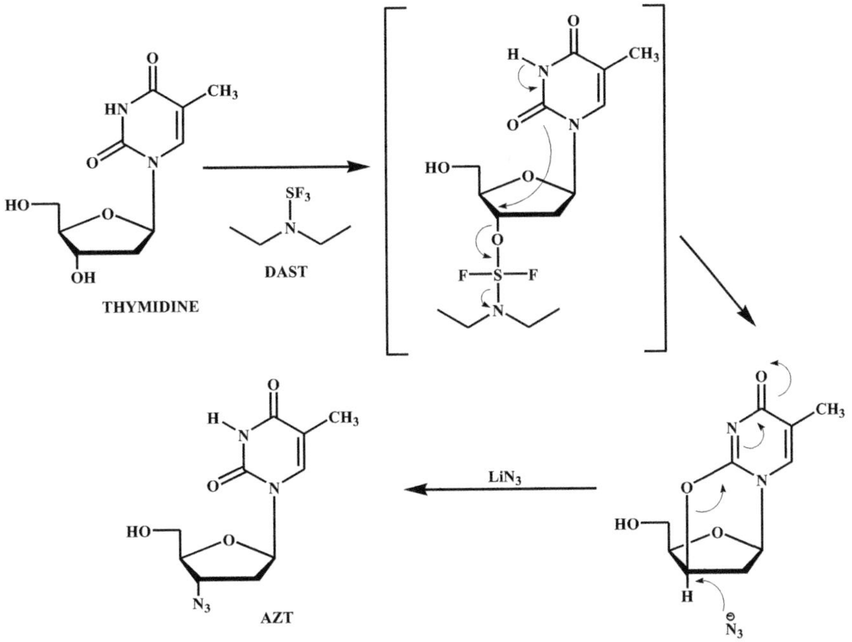

SCHEME 1.1 Synthesis of AZT.[29]

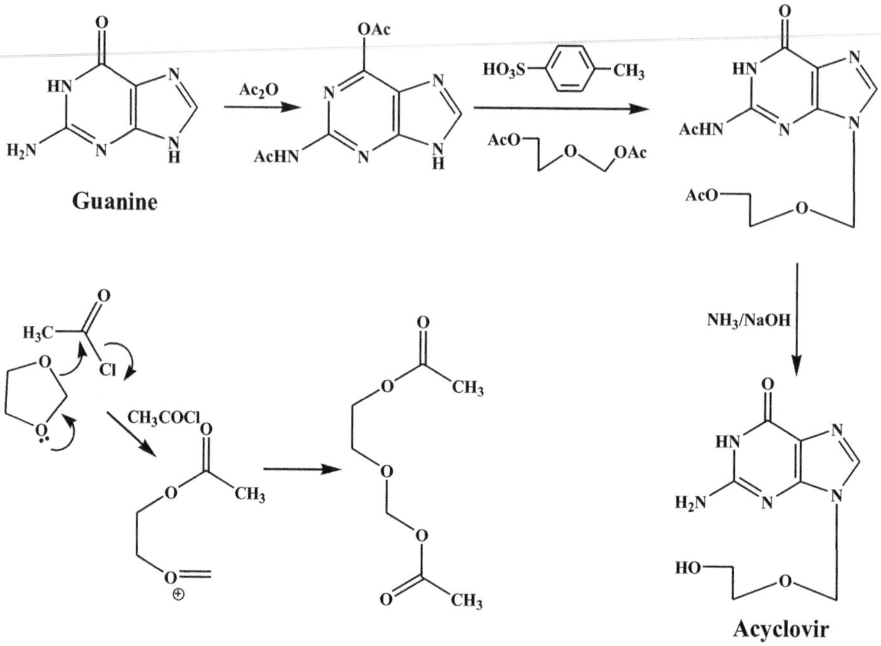

SCHEME 1.2   Synthesis of acyclovir.

Acyclovir, a reverse transcriptase inhibitor, has a mechanism of antiviral activity similar to AZT. The synthesis of acyclovir is shown in Scheme 1.2.

1.4 SYNTHESIS OF PYRIMIDINES AND PURINES

Methods for the synthesis of pyrimidines, purines, and nucleotides are shown in Schemes 1.3–1.7.[30]

Synthesis of pyrimidines

X = H, NH$_2$, OR, SR, NR$_1$R$_2$
Y= Leaving Group; OEt etc.

Examples:

(1)

(2)

(3)

(4)

(5)

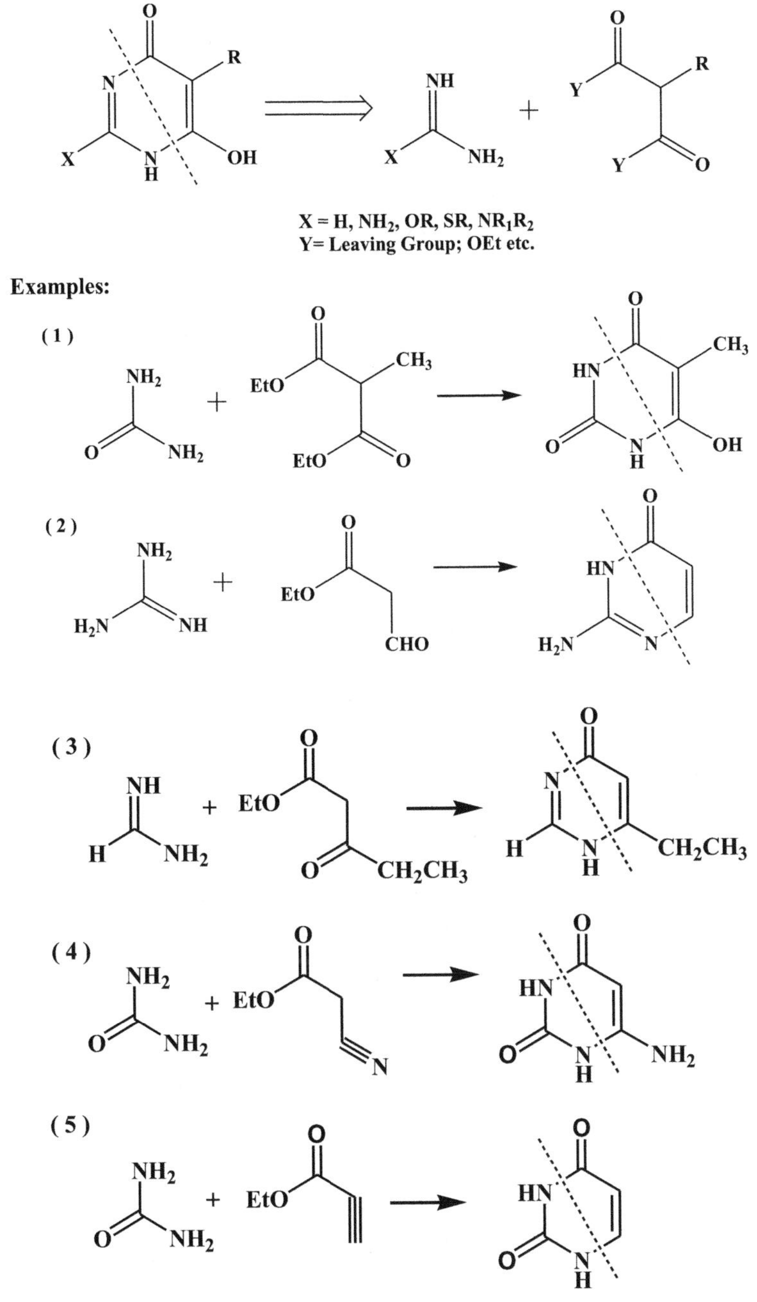

SCHEME 1.3   Synthesis of pyrimidines.

Synthesis of purines

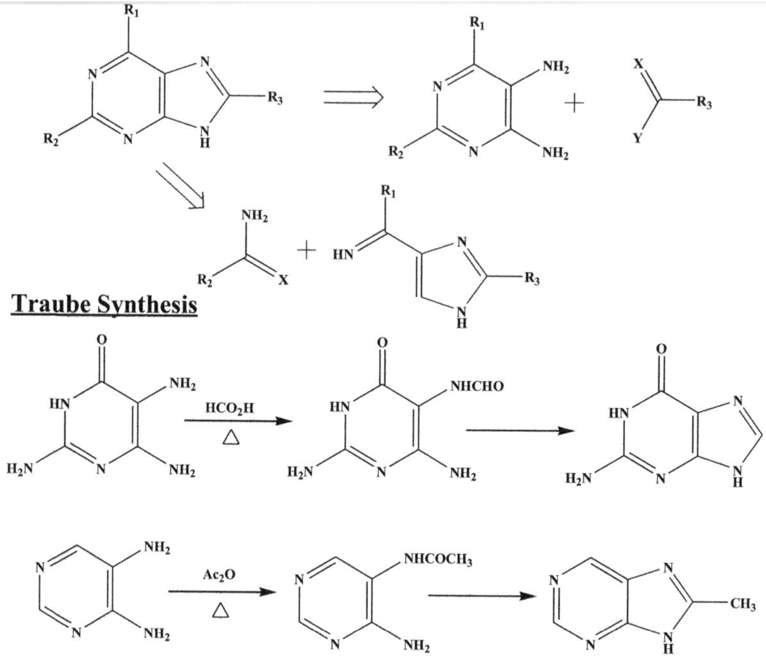

Traube Synthesis

SCHEME 1.4 Synthesis of purines.

Synthesis of purines from pyrimidines

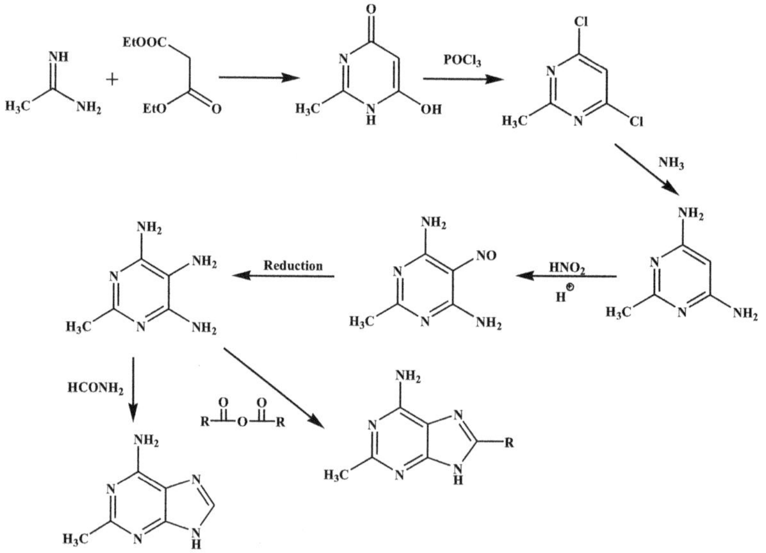

SCHEME 1.5 Synthesis of purines from pyrimidines.

Synthesis of adenine and guanine from uric acid

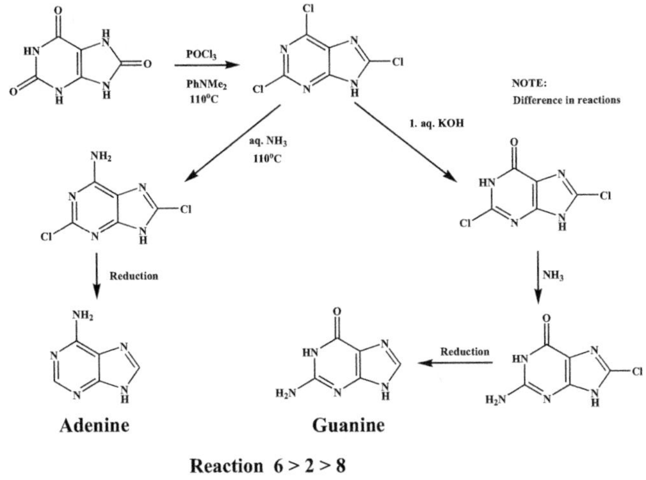

SCHEME 1.6 Synthesis of adenine and guanine from uric acid.

Synthesis of nucleotides

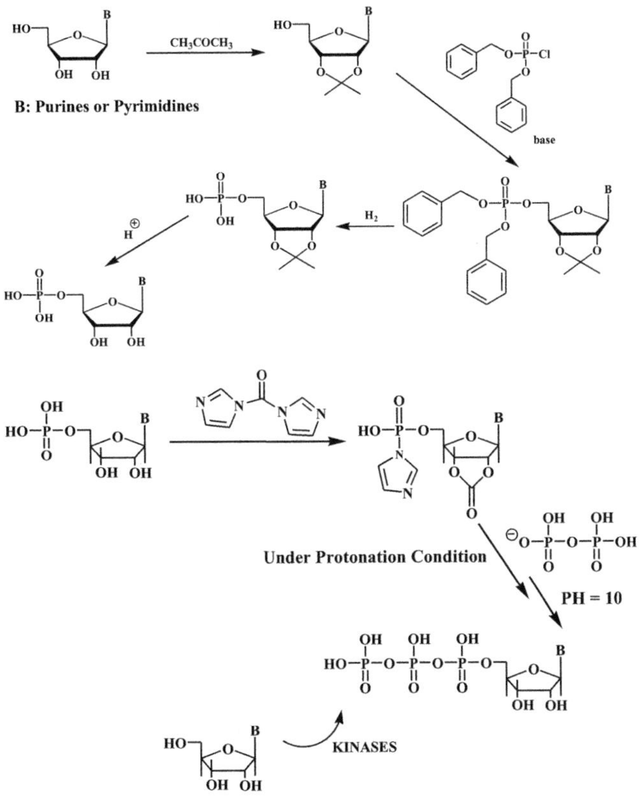

SCHEME 1.7 Synthesis of nucleotides.

1.5 PHARMACOKINETICS

Pharmacological responses can be correlated with the concentration of the drug at the site of action. Pharmacokinetics determine the fate of the drug when administered in animals and humans (Figure 1.13). Since it is difficult to measure the concentration of drugs in several tissues (i.e., brain, liver, heart, lungs), measuring the concentration of drugs in blood is a very good alternative.

1.5.1 ORAL ABSORPTION

When a drug is delivered orally, it crosses the intestinal membrane and then enters the blood supply. The first pass of the drug is through the liver, where metabolism occurs prior to general circulation. The drug and its metabolites are then distributed to various tissues. Finally, the residual drug and metabolites are excreted through the kidneys/bile (Figure 1.14). Ideally, one would like to use drugs orally once or twice a day, and therefore the drug should have an appropriate half-life that can be measured in the blood and metabolites that can be detected in the blood/urine. Too short a half-life will require frequent delivery of the drug, which is not practical, and a long half-life indicates the drug is likely to be highly protein-bound and show toxicity. Following the guidelines of Lipinski's rule and understanding the metabolic profile, one should be able to address these issues. In addition to oral delivery of drugs, the parenteral route, which involves intravenous (IV), intramuscular (IM), intranasal or intrathecal administration, is also commonly used.

A brief summary of the fate of a drug when administered to animals/humans is presented in Figure 1.14.[31]

1.5.2 DRUG METABOLISM

When a foreign protein enters the body, the immune system produces antibodies to neutralize its effect. Small-molecule foreign substances such as drugs are also

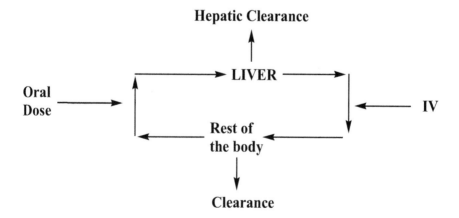

FIGURE 1.13 Fate of drug in vivo.

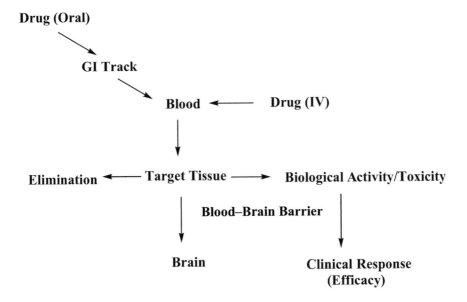

FIGURE 1.14 Routes of drug administration.

metabolized in the liver and eliminated. However, when the foreign substance is a drug, balance has to be achieved for absorption, metabolism and elimination to optimize activity. An understanding of drug metabolism is essential for optimizing activity and safety. Nonpolar (fat-soluble) drugs usually have a longer half-life and will likely show toxicity and therefore are converted to polar and water-soluble metabolites, which are then excreted from the body. Structures of metabolites are determined using radiolabeled drugs, which are usually labeled with ^{14}C or ^{3}H. For safety considerations, incorporation of radioactivity in a drug candidate should be carried out toward the end of its synthesis. As ^{3}H can get exchanged, ^{14}C-labeled compounds are preferred for drug metabolism studies. Specific radioactivity is a measure of radioactivity per mole of compound. Radioactivity is measured in urine/feces. Isolation of metabolites will be done using HPLC, with determination of structures using MS and NMR; ^{14}C and ^{3}H are weak β-emitters. Naturally occurring drugs such as antibiotics can be radiolabeled by biosynthetic incorporation of radioactive precursors.

Metabolites can be toxic, and their formation can be species-dependent. Very rarely are racemates used as drugs because it is possible that one of the enantiomers may get metabolized faster than the other, which could result in buildup of the undesired and toxic enantiomer. There are also examples wherein metabolites may be more promising as drugs than the original drug; for example, Clarinex is a metabolite of Claritin and Allegra is a metabolite of Seldane. When metabolism of a drug creates a new chiral center, its development may be problematic but can also offer new possibilities. The discovery of the successfully used antifungal agent posaconazole is a case in point.

A few examples of the incorporation of radioactive isotopes into drugs are shown in Figure 1.15. Penicillin G labeled with ^{14}C can be prepared by biosynthetic

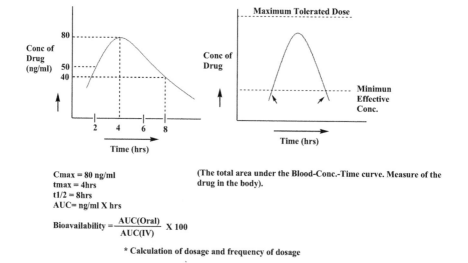

FIGURE 1.15   Synthesis of radiolabeled compounds.

Conc of Drug (ng/ml)

80
50
40

2   4   6   8

Time (hrs)

Conc of Drug

Maximum Tolerated Dose

Minimun Effective Conc.

Time (hrs)

Cmax = 80 ng/ml
tmax = 4hrs
t1/2 = 8hrs
AUC= ng/ml X hrs

(The total area under the Blood-Conc.-Time curve. Measure of the drug in the body).

$$\text{Bioavailability} = \frac{AUC(Oral)}{AUC(IV)} \times 100$$

* Calculation of dosage and frequency of dosage

FIGURE 1.16   Drug bioavailability.

incorporation of ^{14}C-labeled phenylacetic acid, a phenolic group can be converted to radioactive methyl ether by alkylation using ^{14}CH$_3$I, and a carbonyl group can be reduced using NaB^{3}H$_4$, yielding a tritium-labeled drug.

When a drug is administered to an animal and blood samples analyzed over a period of time, the curves showing the blood level of the drug against time can appear as shown in Figure 1.16.

One can derive important information from these graphs, including Cmax (highest concentration of blood level), tmax (time to reach highest concentration of blood

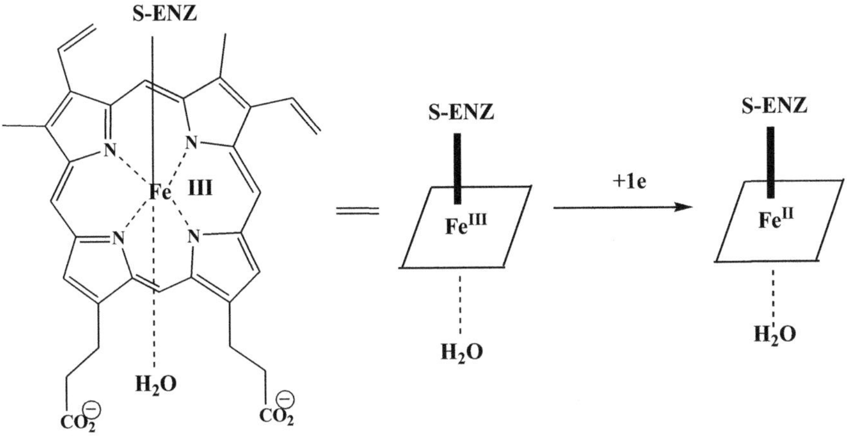

FIGURE 1.17 Active site of cytochrome P450 enzyme containing heme iron center.

level), $t_{1/2}$ (duration of time to maintain half the concentration of the maximum concentration of blood level), and area under the curve (AUC).

Monooxygenation reactions are of major significance in drug metabolism. The most important member of this class is Cytochrome P450, which represents a large group of enzymes belonging to heme-coupled monooxygenases. Cytochrome P450 (CYP) enzymes are encoded by the *CYP* genes. Most important for drug metabolism are the subfamilies of P450 (e.g., 1A, 2A, 3A, 2B, 3A3, 2C19, 2D6, 3A4). These enzymes are so named because they contain a heme cofactor, which upon treatment with carbon monoxide gives a characteristic absorbance at 450 nm. In humans, oxidative metabolism mainly involves CYP 3A4 and CYP 2D6 (Figure 1.17).

Nicotinamide adenine dinucleotide (NAD) is the coenzyme involved in the oxidation-reduction mechanism. NAD participates in hydrogen transfer reactions. The reduction is carried out when a substrate binds to the enzyme by the reductase subunit of the enzyme.

Schemes 1.8–1.10 represent in chemical terms how metabolic oxidation—for example, conversion of R-H to R-OH—takes place. R represents the structure of the drug molecule.

1.5.3 EXAMPLES OF DRUG METABOLISM

Benzene to Phenol

The same principle can be applied as follows for the conversion of aromatic rings to phenols.

In the following pathway, the aromatic ring is oxidized to an epoxide, which can rearrange further to the corresponding phenol. Alternatively, the epoxide ring can be opened via a nucleophilic attack by DNA or an essential protein, resulting in toxicity.

If the aromatic ring in a drug molecule is substituted with an electron donating group, the oxidation process will be facilitated in the ortho or para position. This

$$R\text{-}H \longrightarrow R\text{-}OH$$

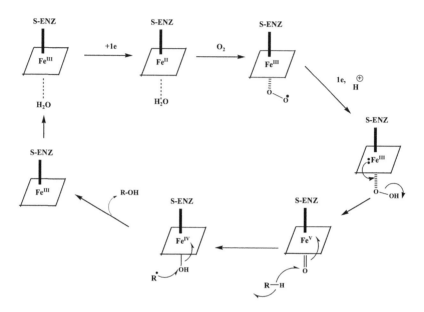

SCHEME 1.8 Conversion of R-H to R-OH.

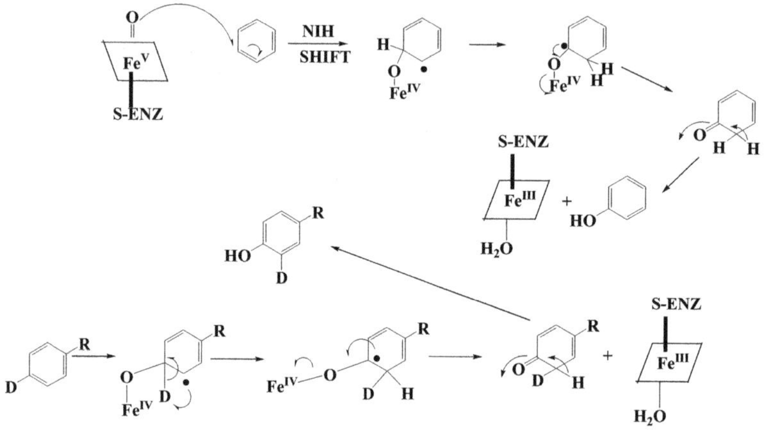

SCHEME 1.9 Conversion of benzene to phenol via NIH shift.

outcome, if detrimental to the development of the drug, can be overcome by substituting the aforementioned positions in the drug molecule with F, Cl, or Br. Many clinically used drugs contain these substituents without losing their biological activities.

The drug probenecid does not undergo aromatic hydroxylation because it has electron withdrawing groups rather than electron donating groups. The arrows in

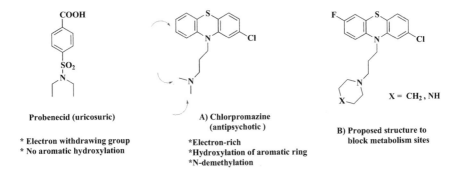

SCHEME 1.10 Epoxidation of aromatic ring and nucleophilic attack.

Probenecid (uricosuric)

* Electron withdrawing group
* No aromatic hydroxylation

A) Chlorpromazine
(antipsychotic)

*Electron-rich
*Hydroxylation of aromatic ring
*N-demethylation

B) Proposed structure to
block metabolism sites

X = CH₂, NH

FIGURE 1.18 Structure of probenecid and chlorpromazine.

Figure 1.18 indicate the sites of metabolism of chlorpromazine, which include aromatic hydroxylation and oxidative N-demethylation.

If the aromatic ring in chlorpromazine is substituted at the hydroxylation site with a fluorine atom, the hydroxy metabolism can be overcome and the rate of metabolism of the N-methyl groups can be modulated by incorporating a piperazine or piperidine ring in its place (Figure 1.18B).

General oxidative metabolic pathways for hydrocarbons and the mechanisms involved are shown in Scheme 1.11.

Oxidative demethylation of aromatic methyl ether follows a pathway similar to that just outlined for the conversion of R-H to R-OH. If one needs to overcome this problem in the development of a drug, $-OCH_3$ can generally be replaced with $-OCF_3$ without loss of activity. Allegra, a metabolite of Seldane, is a more potent antihistamine than Seldane (Scheme 1.12).

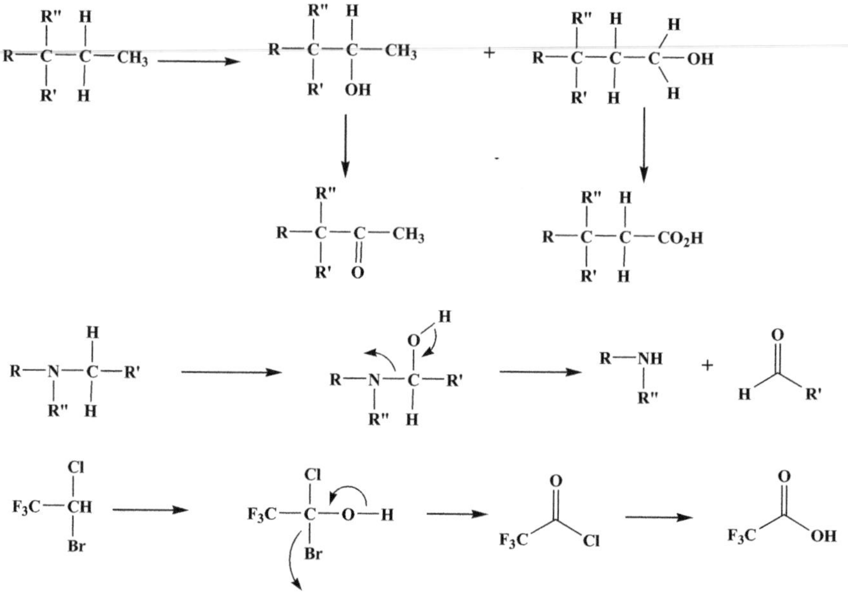

SCHEME 1.11   Metabolism to ketone, amine, and carboxylic acid.

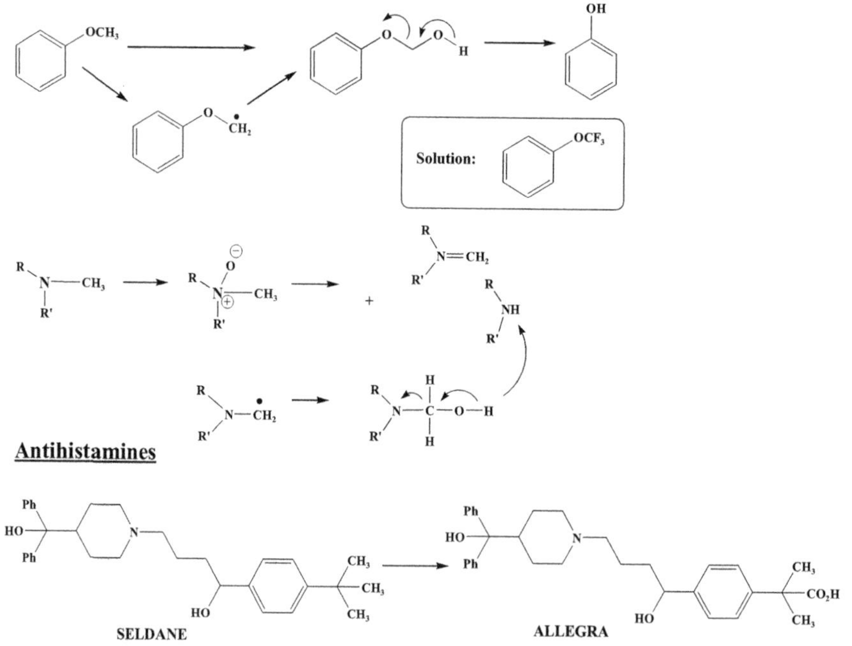

Antihistamines

SELDANE   ALLEGRA

SCHEME 1.12   Oxidative demethylation and metabolism of Seldane to Allegra.

Shown in Scheme 1.13A–C are the metabolic products of a few clinically used drugs.

The general mechanism involved in N-demethylation and oxidation of a sulfur moiety is shown in Scheme 1.14.

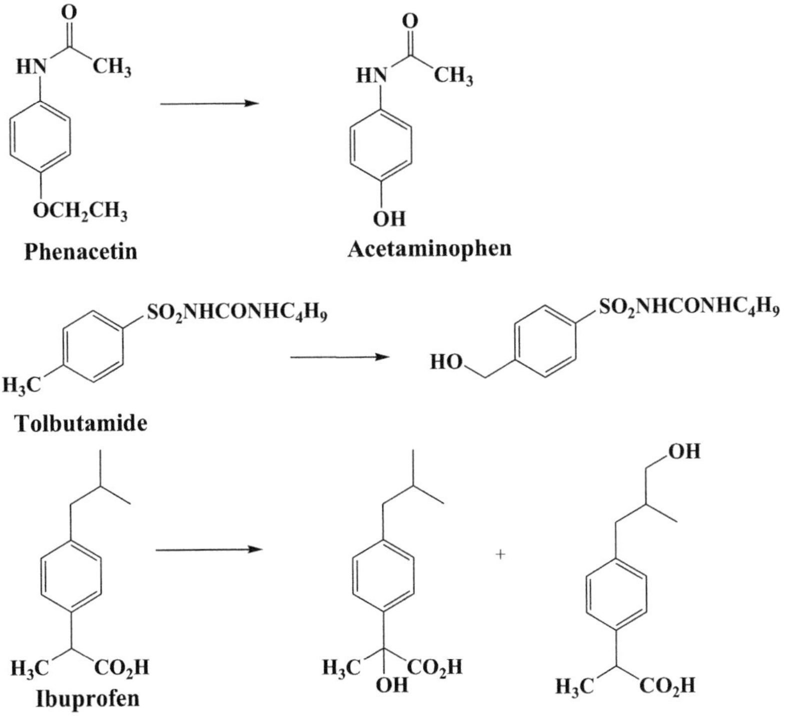

SCHEME 1.13A Mechanisms shown are oxidative dealkylation (Phenacetin), hydroxylation (Tolbutamide, Ibuprofen).

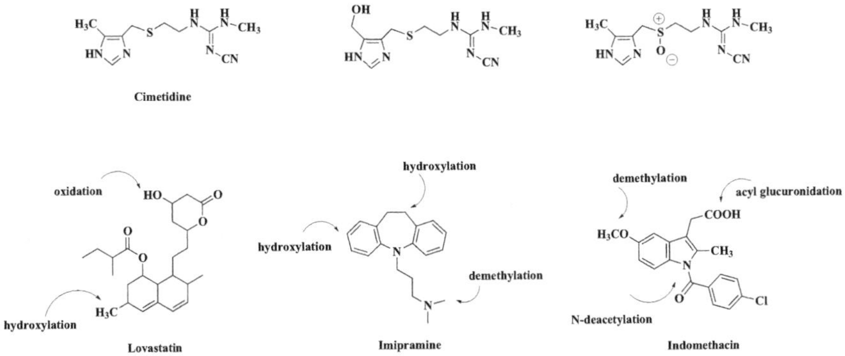

SCHEME 1.13B Mechanisms shown are hydroxylation, N-demethylation, oxidation of sulfur (Cimetidine). Arrows shown in the cases of Lovastatin, Imipramine, Indomethacin) are sites of metabolism.

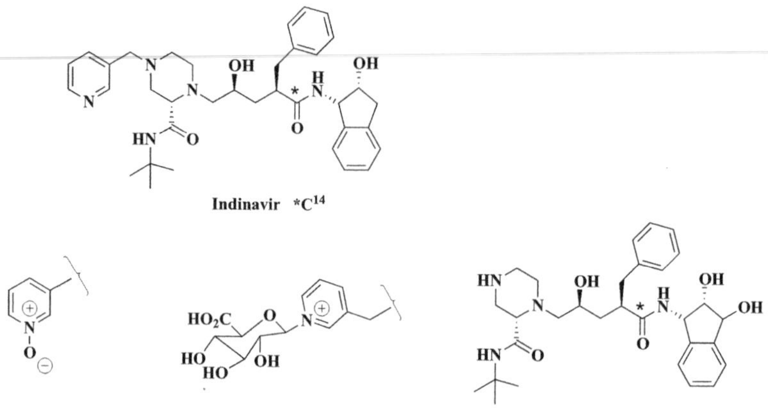

Indinavir $*C^{14}$

SCHEME 1.13C   Metabolism of HIV-1 protease inhibitor indinavir.

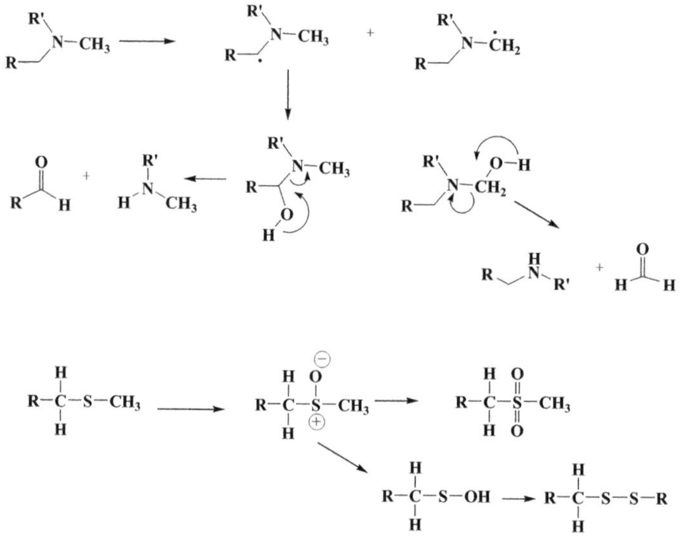

SCHEME 1.14   Mechanism of N-demethylation and metabolism of sulfur-containing groups.

Olefins need to be avoided in a drug, if possible, because they will get oxidized to the corresponding epoxides, which, on principle, could react with DNA or proteins and show toxicity (Scheme 1.15).

Esterases are responsible for the hydrolysis of esters and carbamates. Claritin, for example, is metabolized to an active drug, Clarinex (Scheme 1.16).

Glucuronidation is an important pathway for eliminating a drug or its metabolites (Scheme 1.17). Other pathways for elimination include the transfer of acyl groups by acyl transferases, formation of amino acid conjugates, and sulfation reactions (Schemes 1.18 and 1.19).

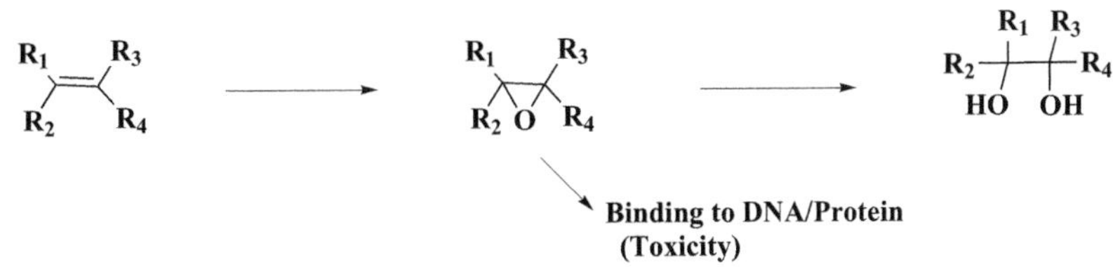

SCHEME 1.15 Metabolism of olefins.

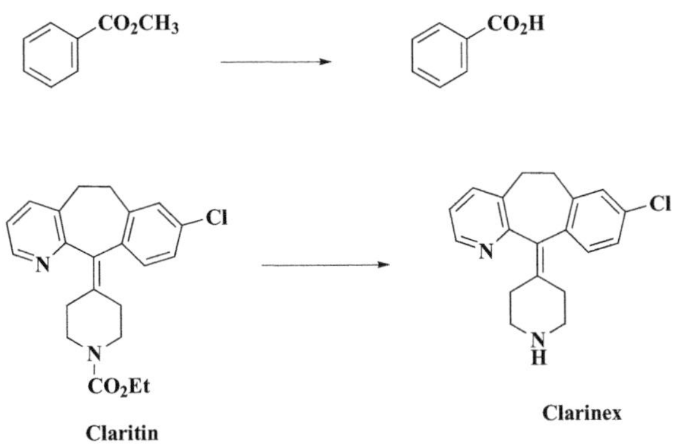

SCHEME 1.16 Metabolism of ester and carbamate groups.

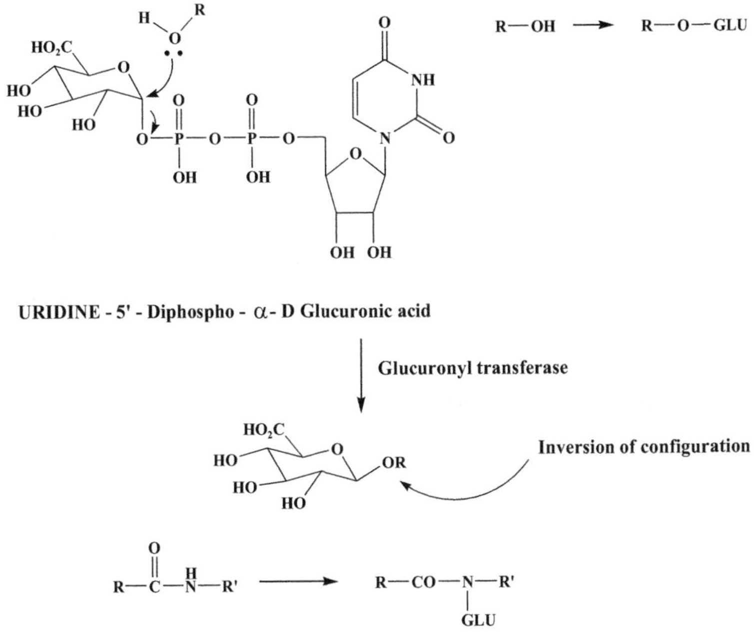

URIDINE - 5' - Diphospho - α- D Glucuronic acid

Glucuronyl transferase

Inversion of configuration

SCHEME 1.17 Glucuronidation of -OH groups.

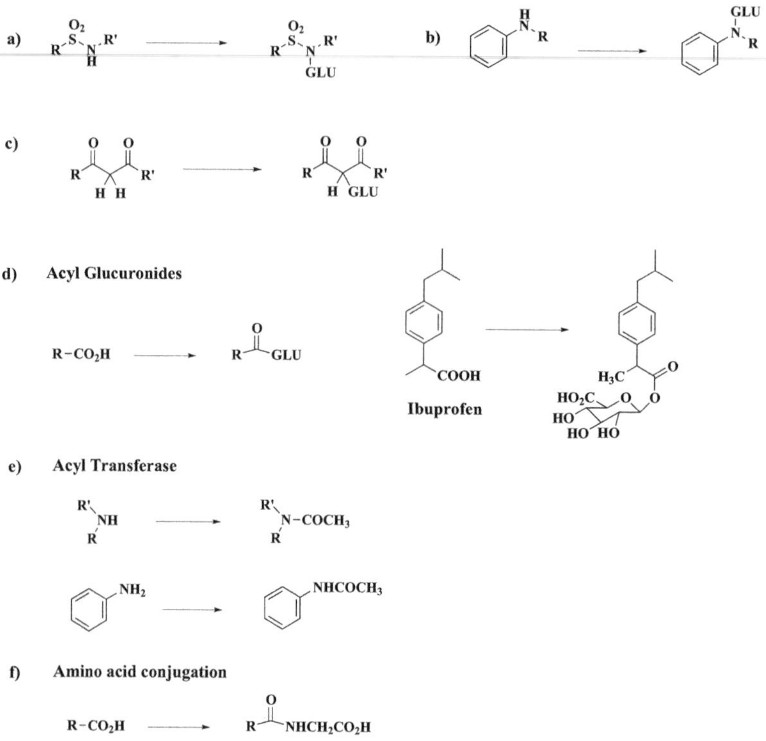
a)
b)
c)
d) Acyl Glucuronides
R-CO2H
Ibuprofen
e) Acyl Transferase
f) Amino acid conjugation
R-CO2H

SCHEME 1.18 Pathways for the elimination of drugs.

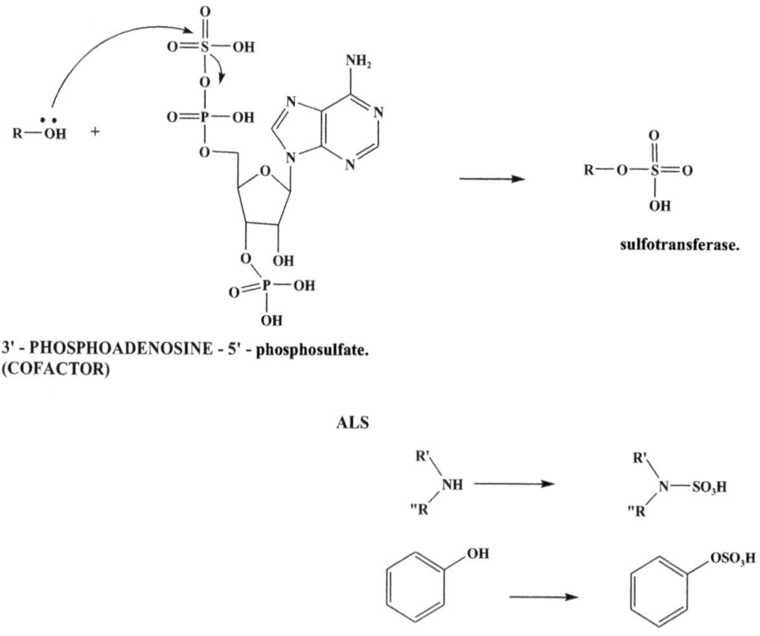
3' - PHOSPHOADENOSINE - 5' - phosphosulfate.
(COFACTOR)
sulfotransferase.
ALS

SCHEME 1.19 Sulfation reactions.

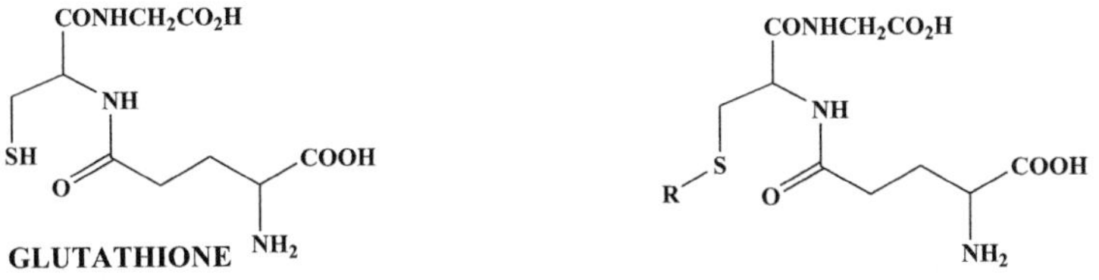

* Acts as a nucleophile (thiol group.)
* Redox

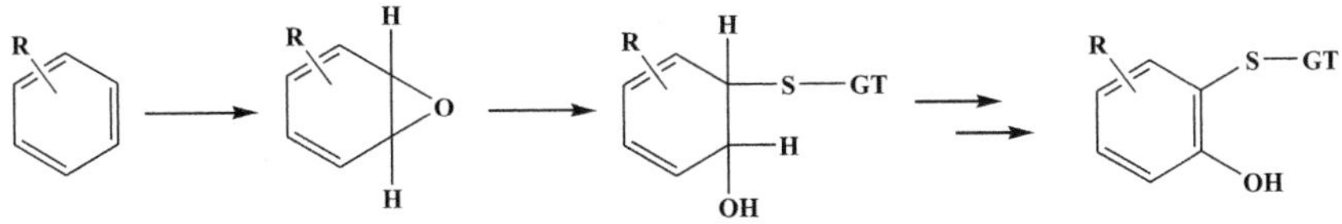

SCHEME 1.20   Formation of glutathione adducts.

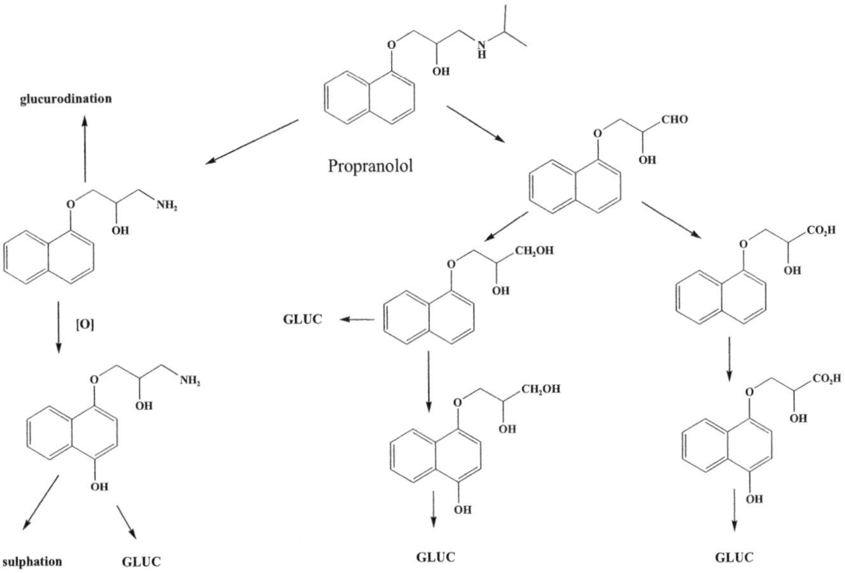

SCHEME 1.21   Metabolism of propranolol.

Glutathione is an important scavenging tripeptide responsible for removing toxic metabolites, and therefore formation of glutathione adducts when a drug is administered to an animal is a sign of toxicity. Glutathione adduct formation signals the presence of reactive metabolites such as epoxides (Scheme 1.20).

A case study showing the metabolism of the drug propranolol, including oxidation of hydrocarbon, demethylation, glucuronic acid derivative and sulfation is given (Scheme 1.21).

REFERENCES

1. Hughes, J. P., Rees, S., Kalindjian, S. B., et al. 2011. Principles of early drug discovery. *Brit. J. Pharmacology* 162(6):1239–1249.
2. Sneader, W. 1985. *Drug Discovery: The Evolution of Modern Medicines*, Wiley, Chichester, New York.
3. Roses, A. 2008. Pharmacogenetics in drug discovery and development: A translational perspective. *Nat. Rev. Drug Discovery* 7:807–817.
4. (a) Piwinski, J. J., Wong, J. K., Green M. J., et al. 1991. Dual antagonists of platelet-activating factor and histamine. Identification of structural requirements for dual activity of N-acyl-4-(5,6-dihydro-11H-benzo[5,6]cyclohepta[1,2-b]pyridin-11-ylidene) piperidines. *J. Med. Chem.* 34(1):457–461. (b) Piwinski, J. J., Wong, J. K., Chan, T. M., et al. 1990. Hydroxylated metabolites of loratadine: An example of conformational diastereomers due to atropisomerism. *J. Org. Chem.* 55(10):3341–3350.
5. (a) Tobert J. A. 2003. Lovastatin and beyond: The history of the HMG-CoA reductase inhibitors. *Nat. Rev. Drug Discovery* 2(7):517–526. (b) Hartman, G. D., Halczenko, W., Duggan, M. E., et al. 1992. 3-Hydroxy-3-methylglutaryl-coenzyme A reductase inhibitors. 9. The synthesis and biological evaluation of novel simvastatin analogs. *J. Med. Chem.* 35:3813–3821.
6. Baumann, K. L., Butler, D. E., Deering, C. F., et al. 1992. The convergent synthesis of CI-981, an optically active, highly potent, tissue selective inhibitor of HMG-CoA reductase. *Tetrahedron Lett.* 33(17):2283–2284.
7. Clader, J. W. 2004. The discovery of Ezetimibe: A view from outside the receptor. *J. Med. Chem.* 47(1):1–9.
8. (a) Cushman, D., and Ondetti, M. A. 1999. Design of angiotensin converting enzyme inhibitors. *Nat. Med.* 5:1110–1112. (b) Cushman, D. W., and Ondetti, M. A. 1991. History of the design of captopril and related inhibitors of angiotensin converting enzyme. *Hypertension* 17(4):589–592.
9. Glushkov, R. G., Adamskaya, E. V., Vosyakova, T. I., et al. 1990. Pathways of synthesis of ranitidine (review). *Pharm. Chem. J.* 24:369–373.
10. Sternbach, L. H. 1979. The benzodiazepine story. *J. Med. Chem.* 22:1–7.
11. Wong, D. T., Perry, K. W., and Bymaster, F. P. 2005. The discovery of fluoxetine hydrochloride (Prozac). *Nat. Rev. Drug Discovery* 4:764–774.
12. Habeeb, A. G., Praveen Rao, P. N., and Knaus, E. E. 2001. Design and synthesis of celecoxib and rofecoxib analogues as selective cyclooxygenase-2 (COX-2) inhibitors: Replacement of sulfonamide and methylsulfonyl pharmacophores by an azido bioisostere. *J. Med. Chem.* 44(18):3039–3042.
13. Hansen, K. B., Hsiao, Y., Xu, F., et al. 2009. Highly efficient asymmetric synthesis of sitagliptin. *J. Am. Chem. Soc.* 131:8798–8804.
14. Bennett, F., Saksena, A. K., Lovey, R. G., et al. 2006. Hydroxylated analogues of the orally active broad spectrum antifungal, Sch 51048(1), and the discovery of posaconazole [Sch 56592; 2 or (S,S)-5]. *Bioorg. Med. Chem. Lett.* 16:186–190.
15. Adams, S. S. 1987. The discovery of Brufen. *Chem. Br. 23*:1193–1195.
16. Hazlet, S. D. C. 1979. Medicinal chemistry of aspirin and related drugs. *J. Chem. Educ.* 56(5):331–333.
17. Richardson, K. 1996. The discovery of fluconazole. *Contemp. Org. Synth.* 3:125–132.
18. Gregory, W. A., Brittelli, D. R., Wang, C-L. J., et al. 1989. Antibacterials. Synthesis and strucutre-activity studies of 3-Aryl-2-oxooxazolidines. 1. The "B" group. *J. Med. Chem.* 32(8):1673–1681.
19. Nicolaou, K. C., Yang, Z., Liu, J. J., et al. 1994. Total synthesis of Taxol. *Nature* 367:630–634.

20. Baeshen, N. A., Baeshen, M. N., Sheikh, A., et al. 2014. Cell factories for insulin production. *Microb. Cell Fact.* 13:141.
21. Alluri, S. S., and Ganguly, A. K. 2019. Design and synthesis of HIV-1 protease inhibitors. *Frontiers in Clinical Drug Research-HIV*, ed. Atta-ur Rahman, 4:1–33. Bentham Science Publishers.
22. Srikanth, V., Bogen, S. L., Arasappan, A., et al. 2006. Discovery of (1R,5S)-N-[3-Amino-1-(cyclobutylmethyl)-2,3-dioxopropyl]-   3-[2(S)-[[[(1,1-dimethylethyl) amino] carbonyl] amino]-3,3-dimethyl-1-oxobutyl]- 6,6-dimethyl-3-azabicyclo[3.1.0]hexan-2(S)-carboxamide (SCH 503034), a selective, potent, orally bioavailable hepatitis C virus NS3 protease inhibitor: A potential therapeutic agent for the treatment of hepatitis C infection. *J. Med. Chem.* 49:6074–6086.
23. Liu, R., Li, X., and Lam, K. S. 2017. Combinatorial chemistry in drug discovery. *Curr. Opin. Chem. Biol.* 38:117–126.
24. Lipinski, C. A., Lombardo, F., Dominy, B. W., et al. 1997. *Adv. Drug Deliv. Rev.* 23:3–25.
25. Watson, J. D., and Crick, F. H. C. 1953. Molecular structure of nucleic acids: A structure for deoxyribose nucleic acid. *Nature* 171:737–738.
26. (a) Crick, F. 1970. Central dogma of molecular biology. *Nature* 227:561–563. (b) Crick, F. H. 1968. The origin of the genetic code. *J. Mol. Biol.* 38:367–379.
27. Pau, A. K., and George, J. M. 2014. Antiretroviral therapy: Current drugs. *Infect. Dis. Clin. North Am.* 28(3):371–402.
28. Furman, P. A., Fyfe, J. A., St. Clair, M. H., et al. 1986. Phosphorylation of 3'-azido-3'-deoxythymidine and selective interaction of the 5'-triphosphate with human immunodeficiency virus reverse transcriptase. *Proc. Natl. Acad. Sci. U S A* 83(21):8333–8337.
29. Czernecki, S., and Valery, J. M. 1991. An efficient synthesis of 3'-azido- 3'-deoxythymidine (AZT). *Synthesis* 3:239–240.
30. Yadav, M., Kumar, R., and Krishnamurthy, R. 2020. Chemistry of abiotic nucleotide synthesis. *Chem. Rev.* 120:4766–4805.
31. Silverman, R. B. 2004. *The Organic Chemistry of Drug Design and Drug Action*, 2nd ed., Elsevier Academic Press, Cambridge, Chap. 7.

2 Enzyme Inhibitors

Enzymes are macromolecular peptides. In enzyme catalytic processes enzymes (E) form complexes with substrates (S) and then transform the substrates into products (P). Enzymes show absolute specificity (i.e., they bind selectively with substrates). Enzymes also exhibit enantiomeric specificity. Enzyme catalysis proceeds through a tetrahedral transition state, which is stabilized by the oxyanion hole (Figure 2.1).[1]

2.1 ENZYME–SUBSTRATE COMPLEX

A substrate binds to the active site of the enzyme to form an enzyme–substrate (E-S) complex[2] using noncovalent electrostatic interactions (i.e., van der Waals forces, hydrogen bonding, and hydrophobic interactions). Hydrogen bonding and salt linkages provide the strongest attractive forces. Substances that bind to the enzymes and decrease their activity are called enzyme inhibitors. Enzyme inhibition can also involve covalent interactions between enzymes and inhibitors (I), which will likely result in toxicity (Figure 2.2). A few such examples are the formation of E-I complexes by alkylating agents, Michael addition, alkyl halides, bromoketones, and epoxides.

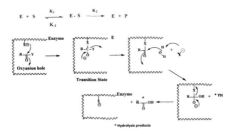

FIGURE 2.1   Generalized enzyme catalysis showing hydrolysis products.

(I) Non-covalent complexes

$$E \ + \ S \ \longrightarrow \ [\text{E-S}] \ \longrightarrow \ P \ + \ E$$

(II) Covalent complexes (toxicity)

$$E \ + \ I \ \longrightarrow \ [\text{E-I}]$$

FIGURE 2.2   Interaction of enzyme with substrate/inhibitor.

DOI: 10.1201/9781003182573-2

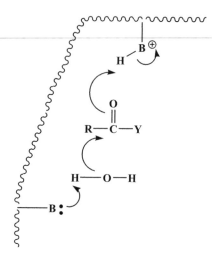

FIGURE 2.3   Simultaneous acid–base enzyme catalysis.

2.2 ENZYME CATALYSIS

Reactions that do not involve catalysts are slow because they involve the formation of unstable positive and negative charges in the transition state, resulting in
higher enthalpy. General acid/base catalysis involves the stabilization of these
charges by proton donation or abstraction. In the case of enzyme catalysis,[3] the
charges in the transition states are stabilized electrostatically by strategically
placed acids, bases, metal ions, or dipoles that are part of the structure of the
enzyme (Figure 2.3).

2.3 MECHANISM OF ENZYMATIC HYDROLYSIS BY PROTEASES

Proteases are a group of enzymes whose catalytic function is to hydrolyze peptide bonds of proteins.[4] They differ in their ability to hydrolyze various peptide
bonds. Serine proteases such as chymotrypsin, trypsin, and elastase perform many
important functions. Serine proteases contain serine in the catalytic domain of the
enzyme. The specificity of enzymatic cleavage is determined by the group at the P1
site (Figure 2.4).

   An example of how serine proteases using a catalytic triad work in the catalytic
domain to hydrolyze the amide bonds in proteins is shown in Scheme 2.1.

   The catalytic triad, which is located at the active site of the enzyme, consists
of three essential amino acids, aspartic acid (Asp102), histidine (His57), and serine
(Ser195), which help to convert the serine hydroxyl group into a nucleophile, which
in turn attacks the carbonyl carbon of the scissile peptide bond of the substrate, generating a tetrahedral transition state. The tetrahedral transition state is additionally

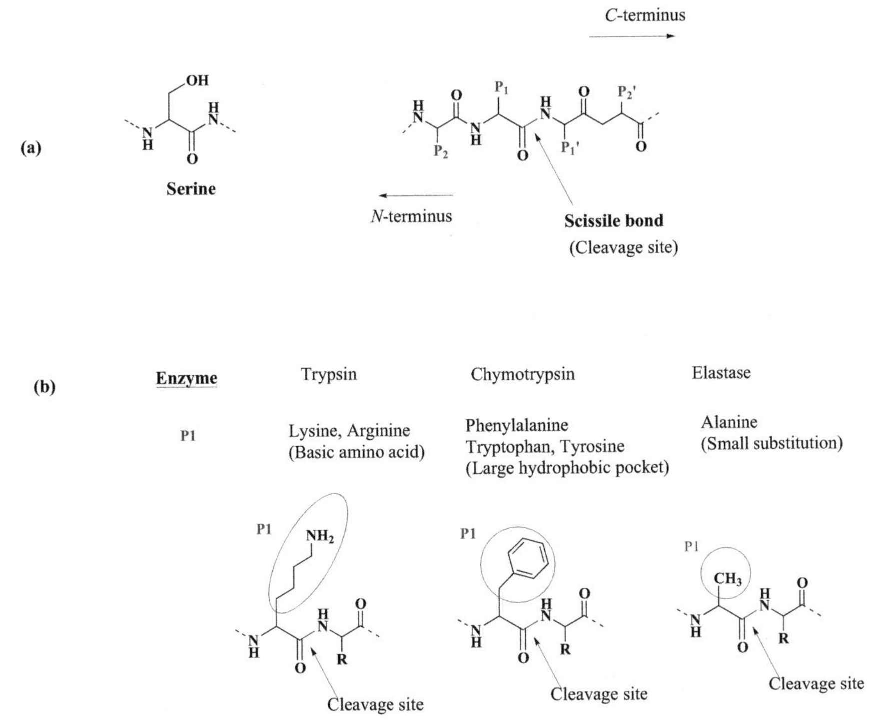

FIGURE 2.4 Serine protease structure, scissile bond, and nomenclature of peptide side chains and different serine proteases and their structures.

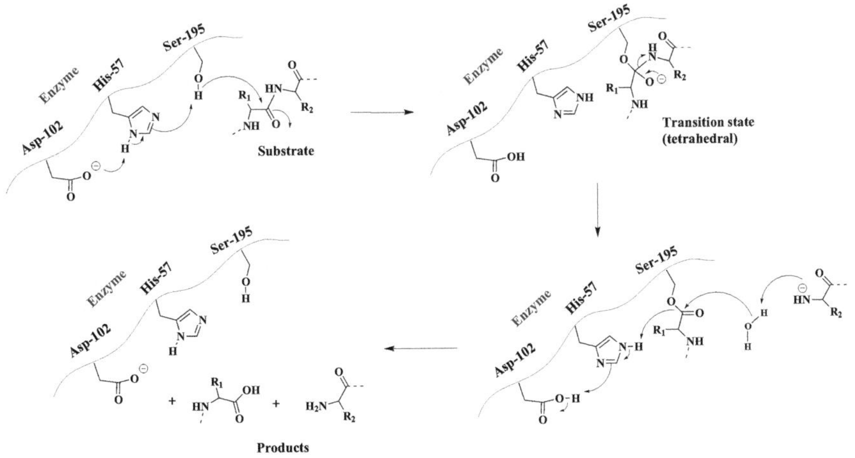

SCHEME 2.1 Catalytic domain of serine proteases (triad).

stabilized by hydrogen bonding of the carbonyl oxygen anion to the backbone NH groups of Ser195 and Gly193, forming the oxyanion hole. The next step is the reconstruction of the carbonyl double bond and the dissociation of the N-terminus of the substrate peptide, generating an acyl enzyme. The nucleophilic attack of water molecules on the acyl enzyme in turn facilitates the cleavage of the C-terminus of the peptide and restores the catalytic triad to its original state. Similarly, aspartic acid proteases use an aspartate residue for catalysis of their peptide substrates, and this will be discussed in the context of the discovery of HIV drugs.

2.4 STRUCTURE OF PROTEINS/ENZYMES

2.4.1 PRIMARY STRUCTURE

Intracellular proteins consist of linear polypeptides. Extracellular proteins usually contain covalent disulfide (-S-S-) cross bridges. This creates loops derived from a single chain or different chains (Figure 2.5).

2.4.2 SECONDARY STRUCTURES

Secondary structures refer to the local spatial arrangement of the main chain atoms without reference to the conformation of the side chain. Local folding of amino acids into stable structures such as α-helices and β-sheets involve hydrogen bonding (Figure 2.6). An α-helix has 3.6 amino acid residues per turn (i.e., amino acid side chains that are three or four residues apart are brought together in space). Each β-sheet is represented by an arrow that defines its direction from N-terminus to C-terminus. Peptide bonds in the β-sheets are planar due to delocalization of the electrons. The β-sheet is parallel when strands point in the same direction or antiparallel when strands point in the opposite direction. A β-hairpin is created when two antiparallel strands are linked by a short loop of two to five amino acid residues.

Myoglobin consists of only α-helices and no β-sheets. Lysozyme and carboxypeptidase consist of both α-helices and β-sheets. An example of an enzyme that has only β-sheets is α- chymotrypsin (Figure 2.7).

FIGURE 2.5 · Disulfide cross bridge.

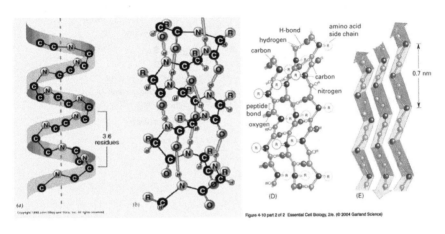

FIGURE 2.6 Secondary structures of proteins.

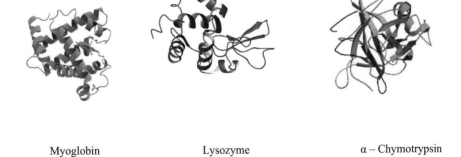

Myoglobin   Lysozyme   α – Chymotrypsin

FIGURE 2.7 Examples of enzymes with α-helices and β-sheets.

2.4.3 TERTIARY STRUCTURES

In the tertiary structures of proteins all the atoms in a single peptide chain are arranged in a complete 3D folding of amino acids. Tertiary structures are stabilized by hydrogen bonds, hydrophobic interactions, van der Waals forces, electrostatic interactions, and disulfide bonds (Figure 2.8).

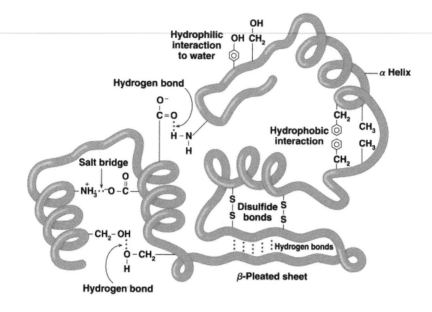

FIGURE 2.8   Tertiary structures of enzymes.

2.4.4 QUATERNARY STRUCTURE

The quaternary structure comprises an association of two or more polypeptide chains to form a complex structure. Thus, many proteins consist of subunits (i.e., α and β subunits). The overall organization of the subunits is known as the quaternary structure. The quaternary structure of the farnesyl protein transferase (FPT) enzyme[6] shows the large active site cavity formed by the interaction of α and β subunits (Figure 2.9). Sarasar fits into this cavity and was advanced up to a phase 2 clinical trial against cancer. However, as an FPT inhibitor, it is now used in the treatment of progeria, a devastating childhood disease.

Enzymes are categorized depending on the type of reaction they catalyze:

1. Oxidoreductases
2. Transferases
3. Hydrolases
4. Lyases
5. Isomerases
6. Ligases

Target-based drug discovery begins with the identification of enzymes or receptors responsible for the biochemical cause of the disease. Inhibitors are designed to block the function of enzymes, and the activity of receptors is accentuated with the help of an agonist or suppressed by an antagonist. For example, angiotensin-converting

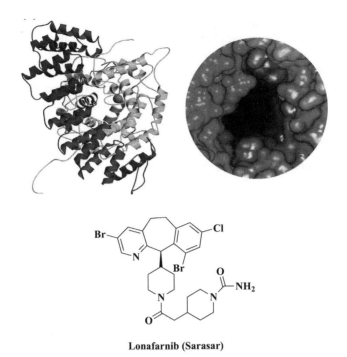

Lonafarnib (Sarasar)

FIGURE 2.9   Active site of the FPT enzyme and structure of Sarasar.

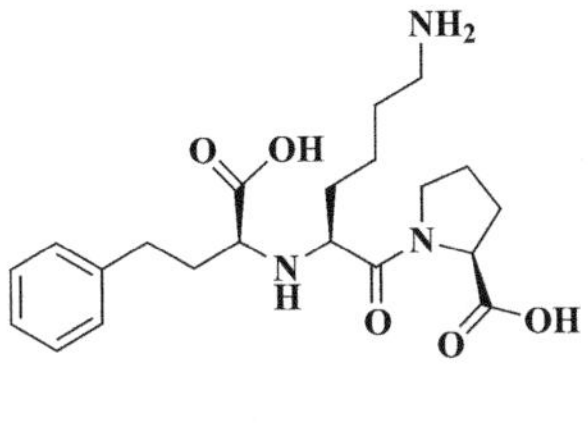

lisinopril (Prinivil)
ACE inhibitor

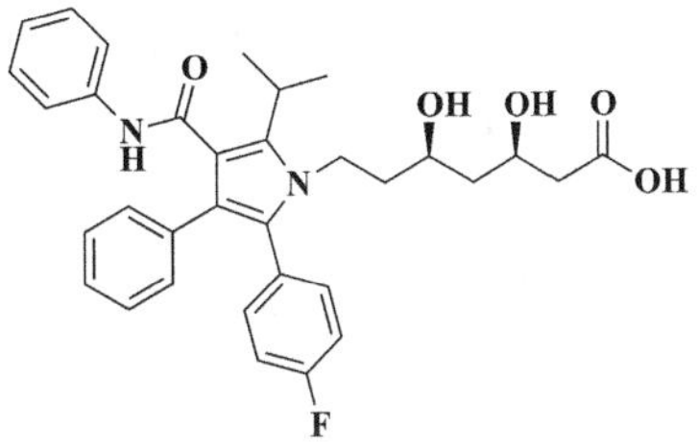

atorvastatin (Lipitor)
HMG-CoA reductase inhibitor

FIGURE 2.10   Examples of enzyme inhibitors.

enzyme (ACE) catalyzes the conversion of angiotensin I to angiotensin II, a potent vasoconstrictor responsible for causing high blood pressure. ACE inhibitors[7] (e.g., lisinopril) treat hypertension by blocking the activity of this enzyme in the renin–angiotensin pathway. HMG-CoA reductase inhibitors[8] (e.g., atorvastatin) are a class of drugs used to lower cholesterol levels by inhibiting the enzyme HMG-CoA reductase, which plays a central role in the production of cholesterol in the liver (Figure 2.10).

With the advent of biotechnology, it has become possible to produce enzymes on a larger scale. Several enzymes have been crystallized and their structures determined using x-ray crystallography. As receptors are, with a few exceptions, generally membrane-bound, they are difficult to crystallize, and hence structural information based on x-ray analysis of the receptors is rarely available. However, receptors can be cloned and assays developed to discover agonists or antagonists.

2.5 ENZYME INHIBITORS

Enzyme inhibitors are discovered via the following sources/pathways:

1. Enzyme inhibitors from natural sources, e.g., antibiotics, antifungals, statins
2. Structure-based enzyme inhibitors, e.g., HIV protease inhibitors
3. Substrate-based enzyme inhibitors, e.g., HCV protease inhibitors
4. Mechanism-based enzyme inhibitors, e.g., FPT inhibitors

2.5.1 ENZYME INHIBITORS FROM NATURAL SOURCES

2.5.1.1 Antibiotics

Prontosil[9] was the first sulfonamide discovered for the treatment of gram-positive bacteria (Figure 2.11). It shows no in vitro activity; however, when administered to an animal it is metabolized in vivo to p-amino benzene sulfonamide, which shows

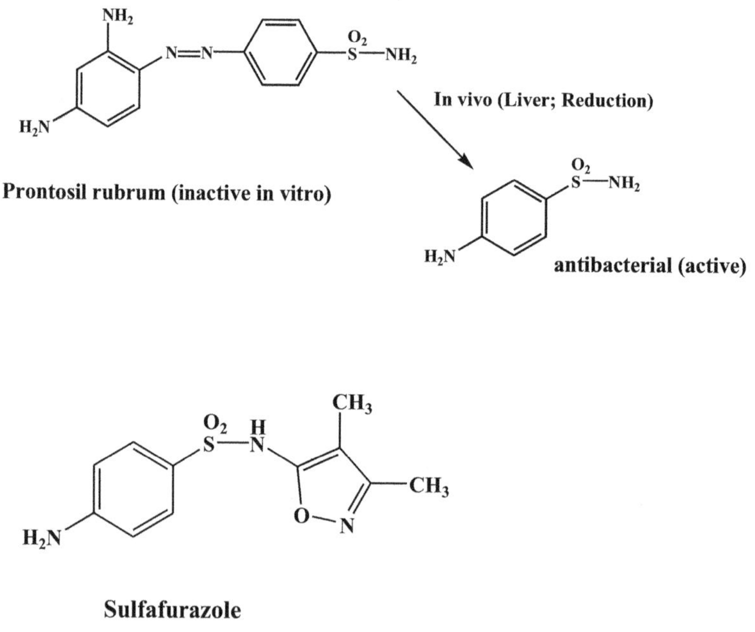

FIGURE 2.11   Examples of sulfonamide drugs.

antimicrobial activity. Many sulfonamide drugs have been discovered and found clinical use. Some of them possess broad-spectrum antimicrobial activity. Sulfafurazole, for example, is a derivative of p-amino benzene sulfonamide that shows broad-spectrum antibacterial activity and has found use as a treatment for urinary tract infection.

Mechanism of Action of Sulfonamides as Antibacterial Agents[10]

Bacteria need tetrahydrofolic acid for purine and pyrimidine synthesis, which in turn is necessary for nucleic acid synthesis. The compound p-aminobenzoic acid is needed for the synthesis of dihydrofolic acid, a precursor of tetrahydrofolic acid. Sulfonamide antibiotics resemble the structure of p-aminobenzoic acid, thus inhibiting the growth of bacteria following the pathway shown in Scheme 2.2.

2.5.1.2 β-Lactam Antibiotics

The discovery of penicillin by Fleming[11] opened an entirely new and perhaps most important chapter in the discovery of life-saving drugs. Members of this class of antibiotics contain a β-lactam ring in their core structure. There are several classes of β-lactam antibiotics, including penicillins, cephalosporins, carbapenems, and penems. Although clavulanic acid is not an antibacterial, being a β-lactamase inhibitor it is widely used along with ampicillin to cure infections caused by bacteria that have developed resistance to ampicillin (Figure 2.12).

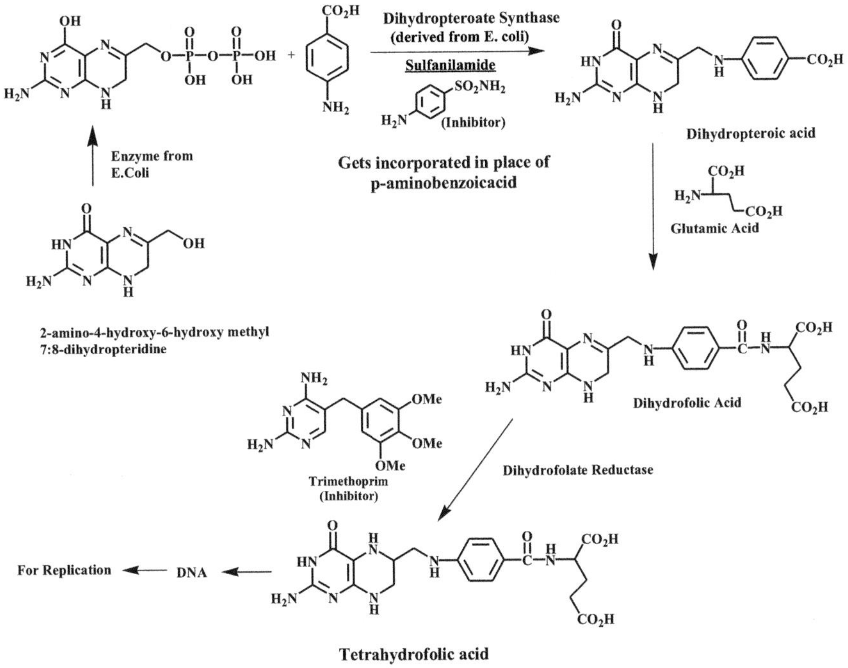

SCHEME 2.2   Biosynthesis of tetrahydrofolic acid.

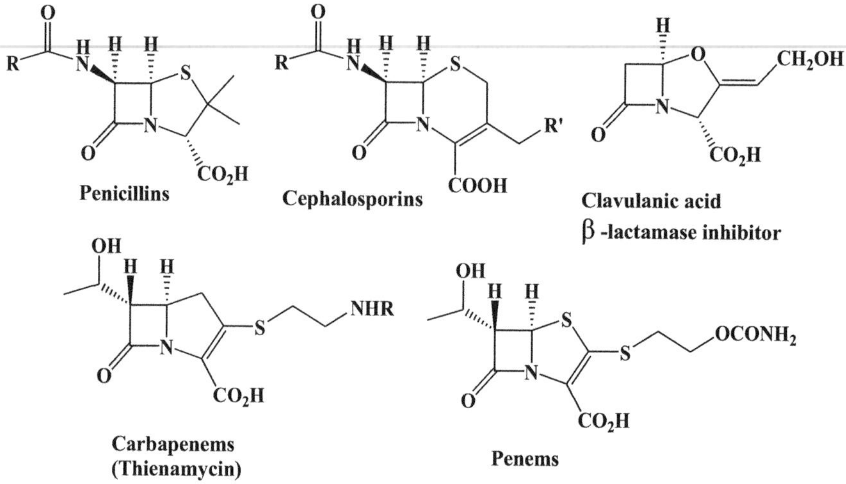

FIGURE 2.12   Examples of β-lactam antibiotics.

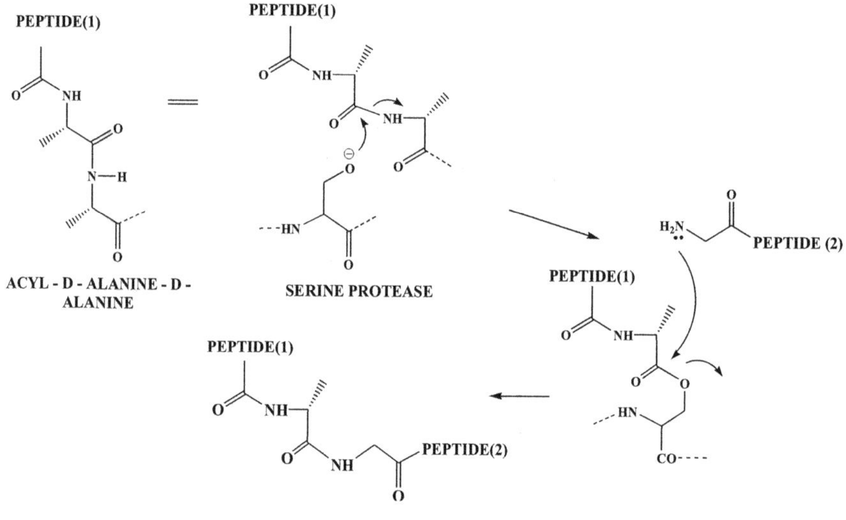

FIGURE 2.13   Bacterial cell wall biosynthesis.

Mechanism of Action of Penicillins and Cephalosporins[12,13]

Penicillins and cephalosporins bind to penicillin-binding proteins and inhibit bacterial cell wall synthesis. Penicillin-binding proteins are involved in cross-linking of the peptidoglycan layer of the cell wall and are essential for bacterial survival (Figure 2.13). Cross linkage involves cleavage of the acyl-D-Ala-D-Ala subunit of peptide 1, and the resulting cleavage intermediate reacts with peptide 2 to form the bacterial cell wall. Penicillins and cephalosporins with the β-lactam ring mimic the

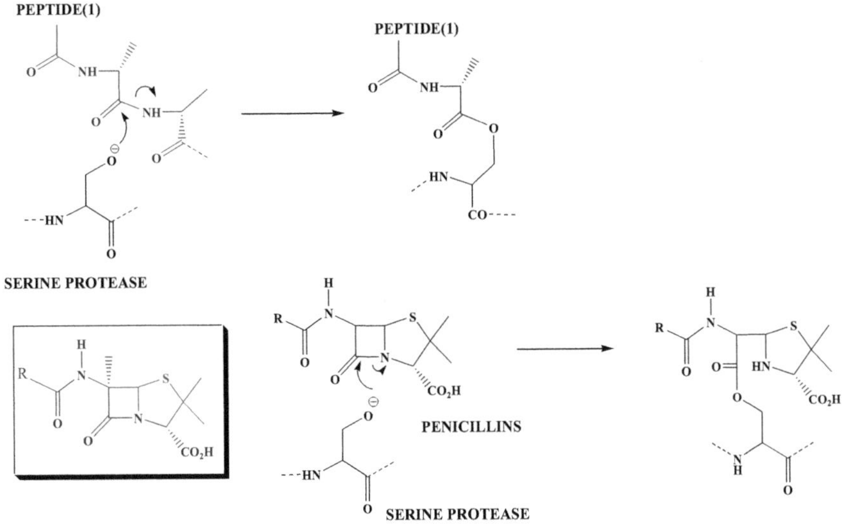

FIGURE 2.14   Inhibition of bacterial cell wall biosynthesis by penicillin.

structure of the acyl-D-Ala-D-Ala of peptide 1 and react preferentially with the serine protease, thus avoiding the cleavage of the acyl -D-Ala-D-Ala residue in the structure of peptide 1 and preventing the growth of the bacterial cell wall (Figure 2.14).

Production of 6-Aminopenicillanic acid (6-APA)
and Penicillins by Fermentation[14]

Fermentation using *Penicillium chrysogenum* in a medium containing corn steep liquor is an important source for the preparation of 6-APA, a crucial starting material for the synthesis of novel synthetic penicillins. In addition, the side chains in penicillins can be incorporated by adding the proper precursors to the fermentation medium, as illustrated in Scheme 2.3 for the preparation of penicillin G and penicillin V.

The synthesis of methicillin and carbenicillin illustrates the general method for the preparation of all clinically used penicillins (Scheme 2.4).

The intermediate 7-aminocephalosporanic acid is important for the synthesis of newer cephalosporins (Scheme 2.5)[14]. In addition, penicillin can be converted to cephalosporin, as shown in Scheme 2.6.

Cephalosporins

Conversion of Penicillin to Cephalosporin[15]

The synthesis of cefamandole and cefmenoxime demonstrates the general method of preparation of clinically used cephalosporins. The structural features responsible for the spectrum of activity/pharmacokinetics of cefmenoxime are shown in Scheme 2.7 using arrows.

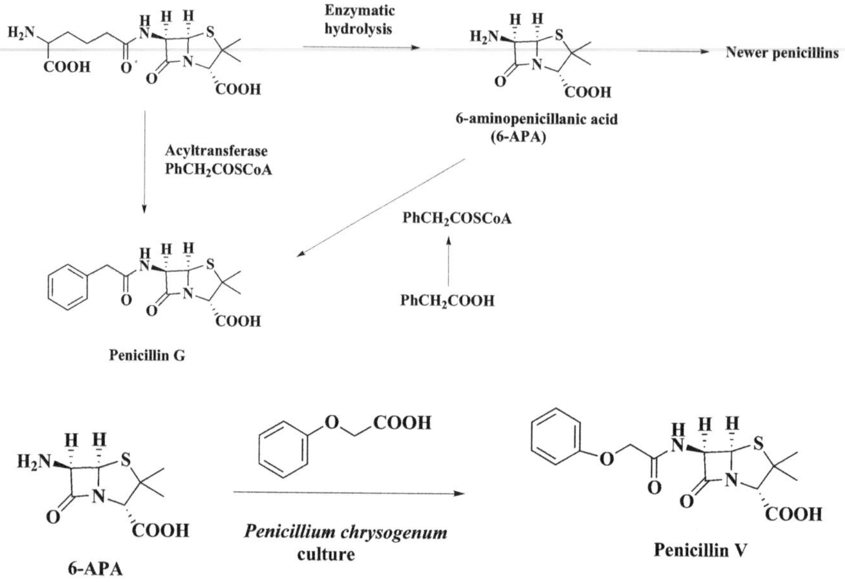

SCHEME 2.3 Synthesis of penicillin antibiotics via 6-APA.

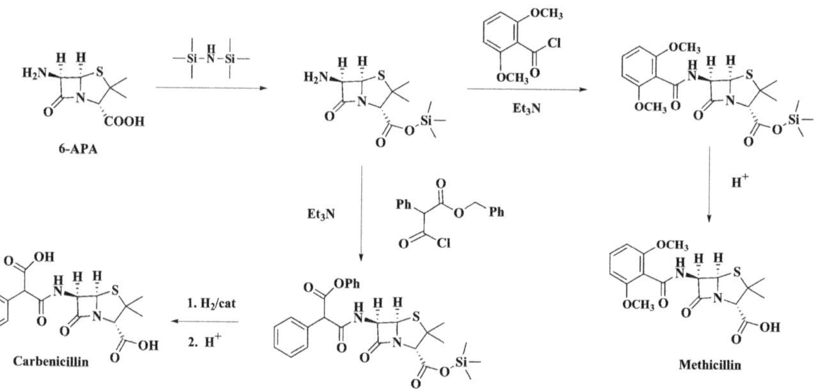

SCHEME 2.4 Synthesis of methicillin and carbenicillin.

2.5.1.3 Macrolide Antibiotics

The most widely used antibiotics of this class include erythromycin and azithromycin. Erythromycin was discovered in 1952 using the fermentation of *Saccharopolyspora erythraea* and has been widely used since its discovery for the treatment of respiratory and skin infections, among other diseases, caused by gram-positive bacteria. It is used orally and considered to be safe, though it can cause gastric irritation and

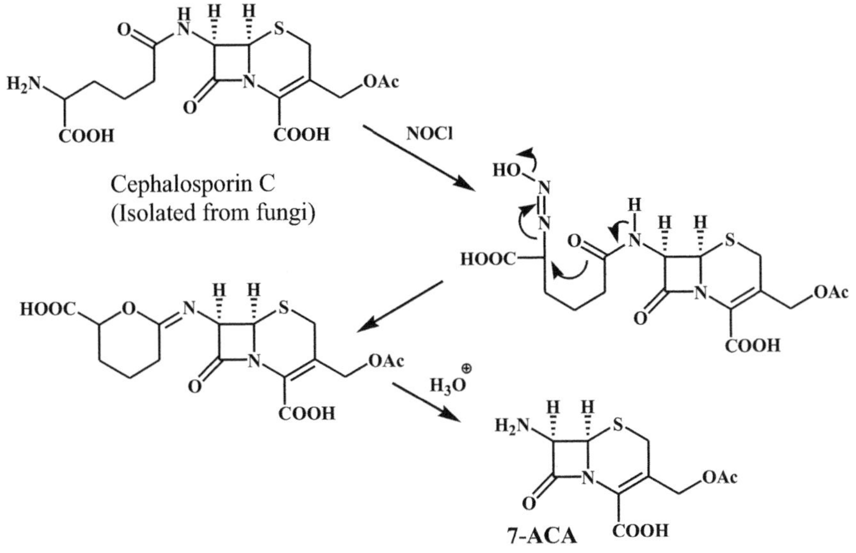

SCHEME 2.5 Preparation of 7-aminocephalosporanic acid (7-ACA).

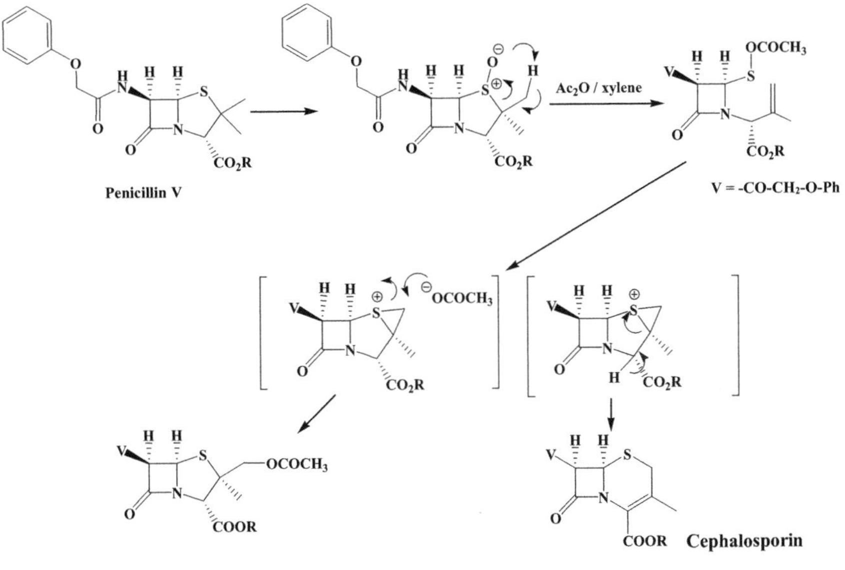

SCHEME 2.6 Conversion of penicillin to cephalosporin by Morin rearrangement.

is also known to be associated with cardiovascular problems. Erythromycin is an inhibitor of the P450 enzyme and thus causes drug–drug interactions and has to be judiciously used when patients are taking other medications. Patients who are allergic to penicillin are recommended to use erythromycin.

(a)

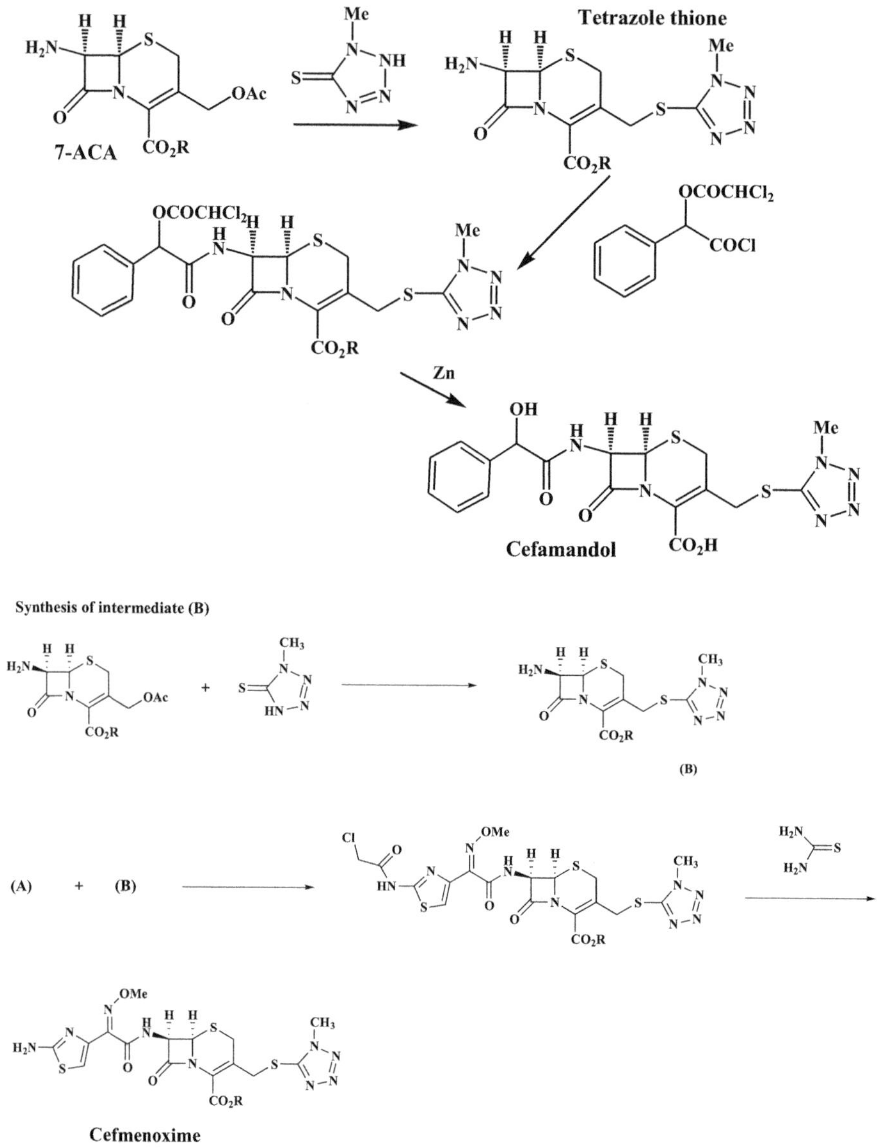

SCHEME 2.7   Synthesis of cefamandole and cefmenoxime.

The second generation of antibiotics in this class that is orally active is represented by azithromycin, which possesses an antibacterial spectrum against gram-
positive organisms that is similar to that seen with erythromycin. In addition, it shows
some gram-negative activity. Overall, the safety profile of azithromycin is superior

to erythromycin; for example, it does not show any cardiovascular side effects and has much less drug–drug interactions. In fact, it has become the drug of choice for treating respiratory infections. Both of these antibiotics have a similar mechanism of action that involves binding to the 50S subunit of the bacterial RNA complex, thus inhibiting protein synthesis. Azithromycin is derived from erythromycin using a Beckmann rearrangement of the oxime, as shown in Scheme 2.8.

2.5.1.4 Antifungals

Azole antifungals[17] are widely used to cure *Candida* infections and those that are more serious and caused by opportunistic fungi such as *Cryptococcus* and *Aspergillus*. The latter category is found more commonly in AIDS and cancer patients.

Ergosterol is required for fungi to survive and is biosynthesized from lanosterol via demethylation at the C14 position (Scheme 2.9). Azole antifungals inhibit this biosynthetic step. Some of the more commonly used antifungals are shown in Figure 2.15, and they all contain either an azole or a triazole ring. Among these, miconazole is used topically, and ketoconazole, fluconazole, and posaconazole are used orally.

The synthesis of miconazole, fluconazole, and ketoconazole is shown in Scheme 2.10.

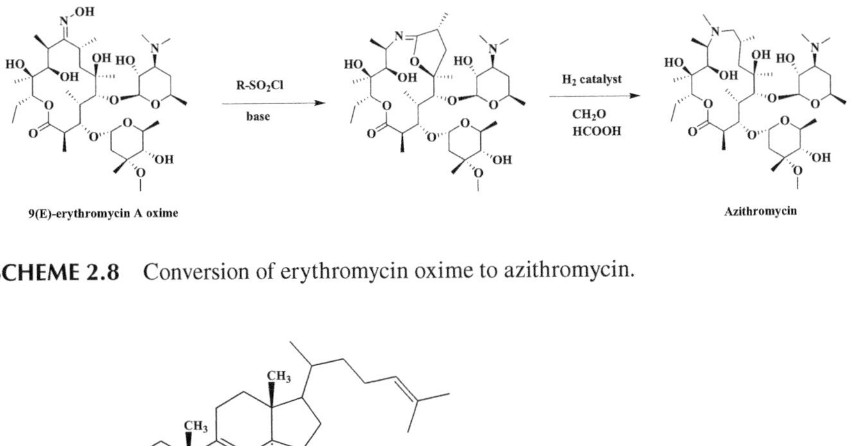

SCHEME 2.8   Conversion of erythromycin oxime to azithromycin.

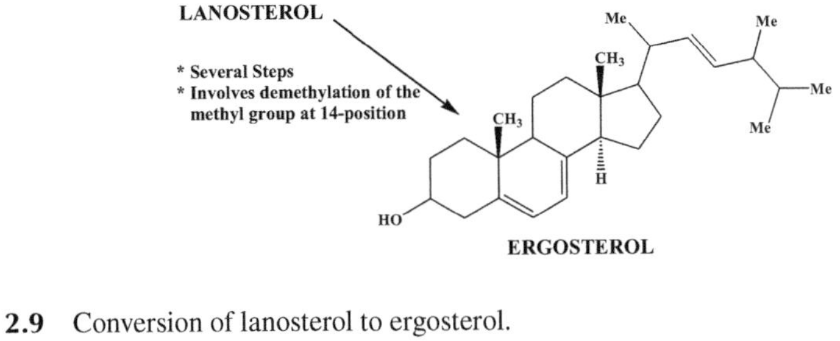

SCHEME 2.9   Conversion of lanosterol to ergosterol.

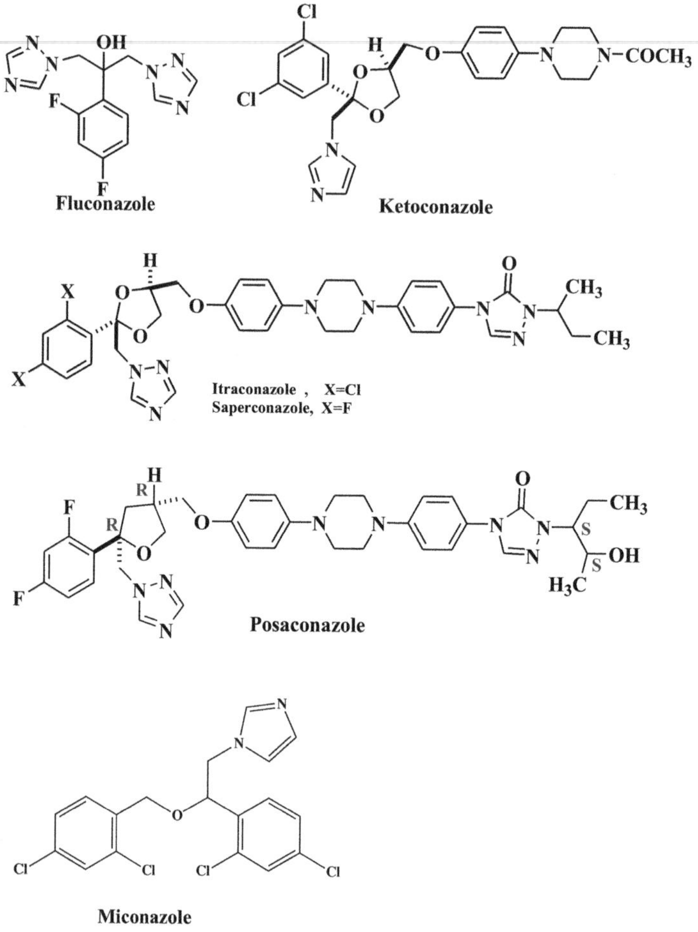

FIGURE 2.15   Structure of azole antifungals.

SCH 51048

Ketoconazole contains the acid labile dioxolane moiety, which was replaced in SCH 51048[18] (Figure 2.16) by a tetrahydrofuran ring to increase the stability of the compound toward an acidic pH.

All possible stereoisomers of the general structure represented by SCH 51048 were synthesized and evaluated for their antifungal activity. SCH 51048 with R,R absolute stereochemistry was found to be most active. Based on its activity and pharmacokinetic properties, including oral absorption, it was advanced further. It was recognized that in vivo SCH 51048 was converted to a more potent mono-hydroxylated metabolite, and using mass spectrometry it was determined that the hydroxylation had occurred at the side chain alkyl group. After synthesizing all the

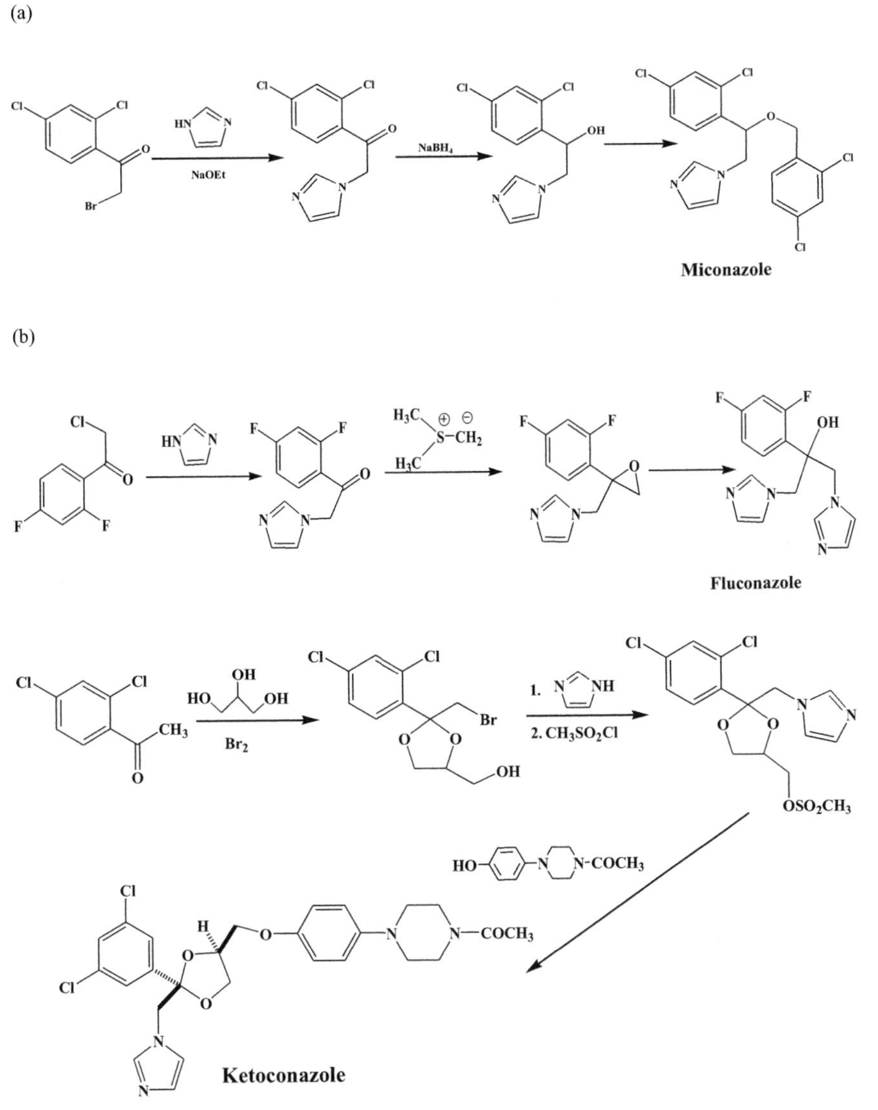

(a)

(b)

SCHEME 2.10   Synthesis of miconazole, fluconazole, and ketoconazole.

possible stereoisomers caused by the hydroxylation of the CH_2 group in the side chain, posaconazole was advanced as the clinical candidate. Based on its superior activity in the clinic, it is now widely used for the treatment of serious fungal diseases caused by opportunistic fungi in cancer and AIDS patients. The synthesis of SCH 51048 and posaconazole shown in Schemes 2.11 and 2.12 demonstrates the importance and power of synthetic organic chemistry in drug discovery. Possible sites of hydroxylation in the structure of the hydroxy metabolite are indicated by arrows in Scheme 2.11.

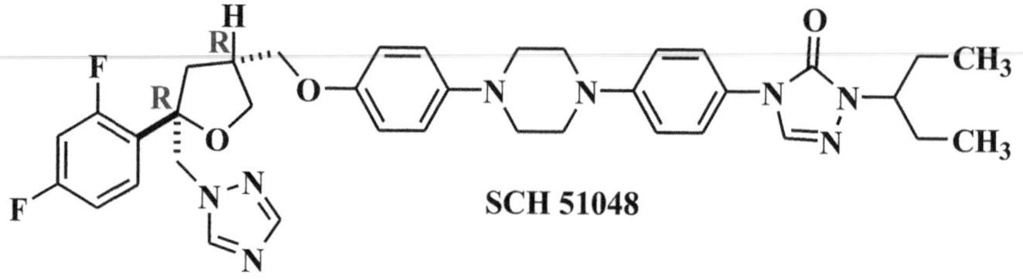

FIGURE 2.16   Structure of SCH 51048.

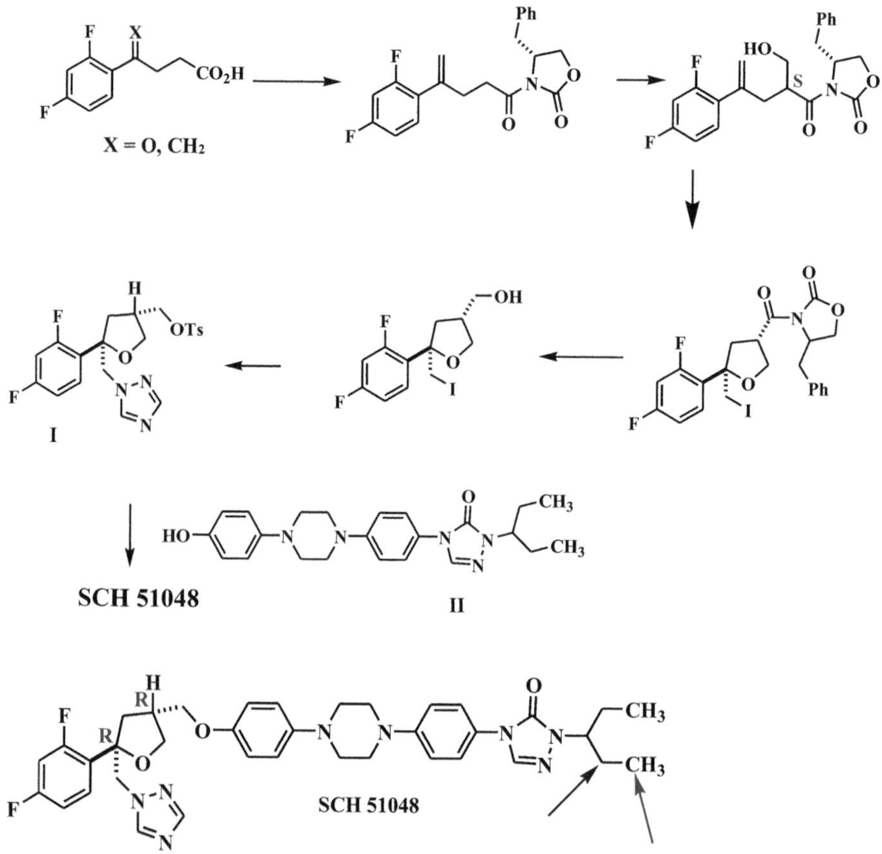

SCHEME 2.11   Synthesis of SCH 51048.

Posaconazole

Posaconazole (Figure 2.17)[19] is a broad-spectrum antifungal that is active against *Aspergillus* species, *Cryptococcus* species, and *Histoplasma* species. Extensive clinical trials also showed posaconazole to be safe, and it is used to treat AIDS and cancer patients. The synthesis of posaconazole is shown in Scheme 2.12.

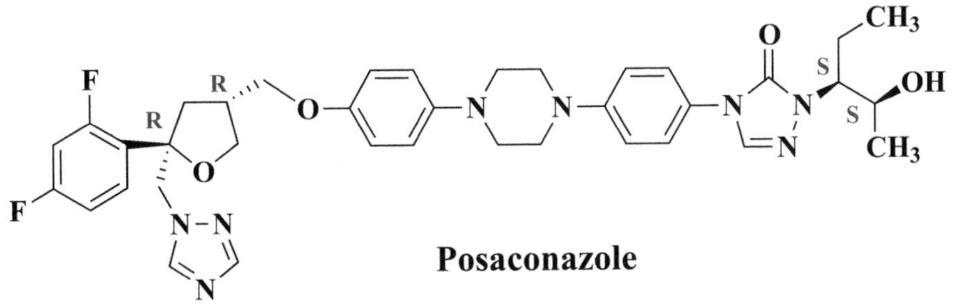

Posaconazole

FIGURE 2.17   Structure of posaconazole.

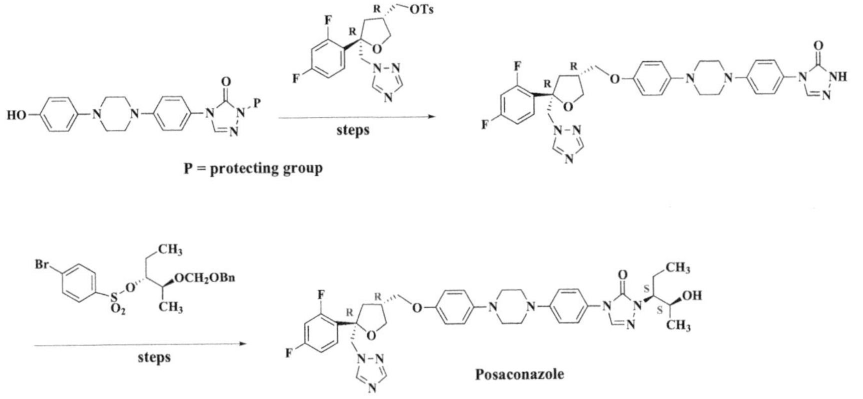

P = protecting group

steps

steps   Posaconazole

SCHEME 2.12   Synthesis of posaconazole.

2.5.1.5 Cholesterol-Lowering Drugs

Coronary artery disease is the leading cause of death in the United States. Atherosclerosis is caused by the buildup of cholesterol (plaque) on the inner walls of arteries. The major source of cholesterol in the human body is the biosynthesis of cholesterol in liver and food. Lipitor, for example, lowers blood cholesterol by inhibiting HMG-CoA reductase in the liver, and Zetia inhibits absorption of cholesterol from food by interfering with cholesterol transporter NPC1L1, which is expressed at the apical surface of enterocytes.

The rate-determining step in the biosynthesis of cholesterol[20] is the formation of mevalonic acid lactone. Statins—that is, lovastatin and atorvastatin (Lipitor) (Figure 2.18)—inhibit HMG-CoA reductase activity, thus inhibiting biosynthesis of mevalonic acid lactone (Scheme 2.13). The synthesis of Lipitor[21] is shown in Scheme 2.14.

The discovery of Zetia[22] began initially as a search for acyl coenzyme A:cholesterol acyltransferase (ACAT) inhibitors, which were implicated in lowering cholesterol levels in hamsters when they were fed a high-cholesterol diet. After extensive studies it was found that monocyclic β-lactams showed the most promise not as ACAT inhibitors but as agents that lowered serum cholesterol in animals fed a

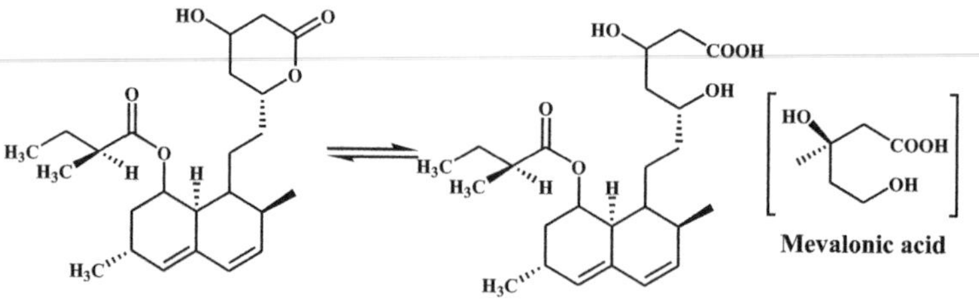

Lovastatin
Natural product (fermentation)
Merck

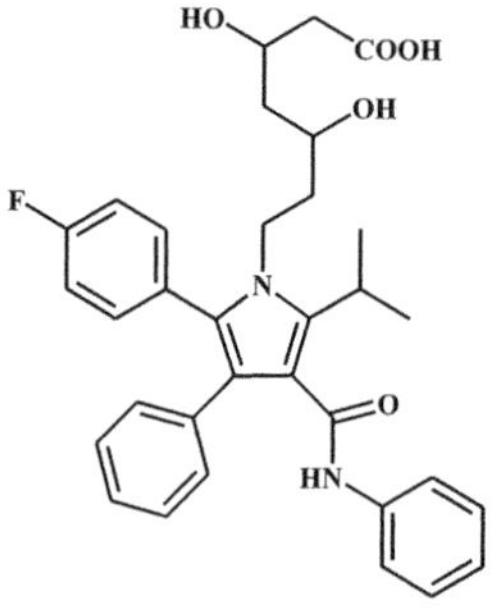

Atorvastatin (Lipitor)
Synthetic
Pfizer (Warner-Lambert)

FIGURE 2.18 Natural and synthetic statins as cholesterol-lowering agents.

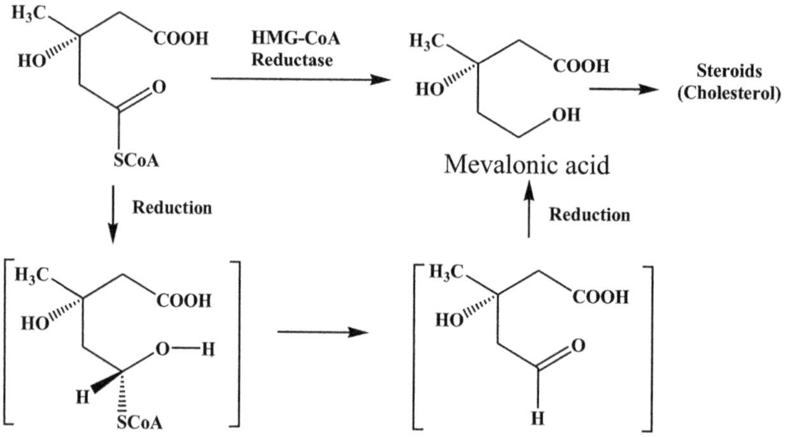

SCHEME 2.13 Mevalonic acid biosynthesis.

high-cholesterol diet. The structure–activity relationship of the analogs synthesized was followed using in vivo tests, which also afforded important clues as to how they were metabolized. Based on all this information, ezetimibe (Zetia) was synthesized and advanced to the clinic, where it was found to be safe and effective in lowering cholesterol. The synthesis of Zetia is shown in Scheme 2.15.

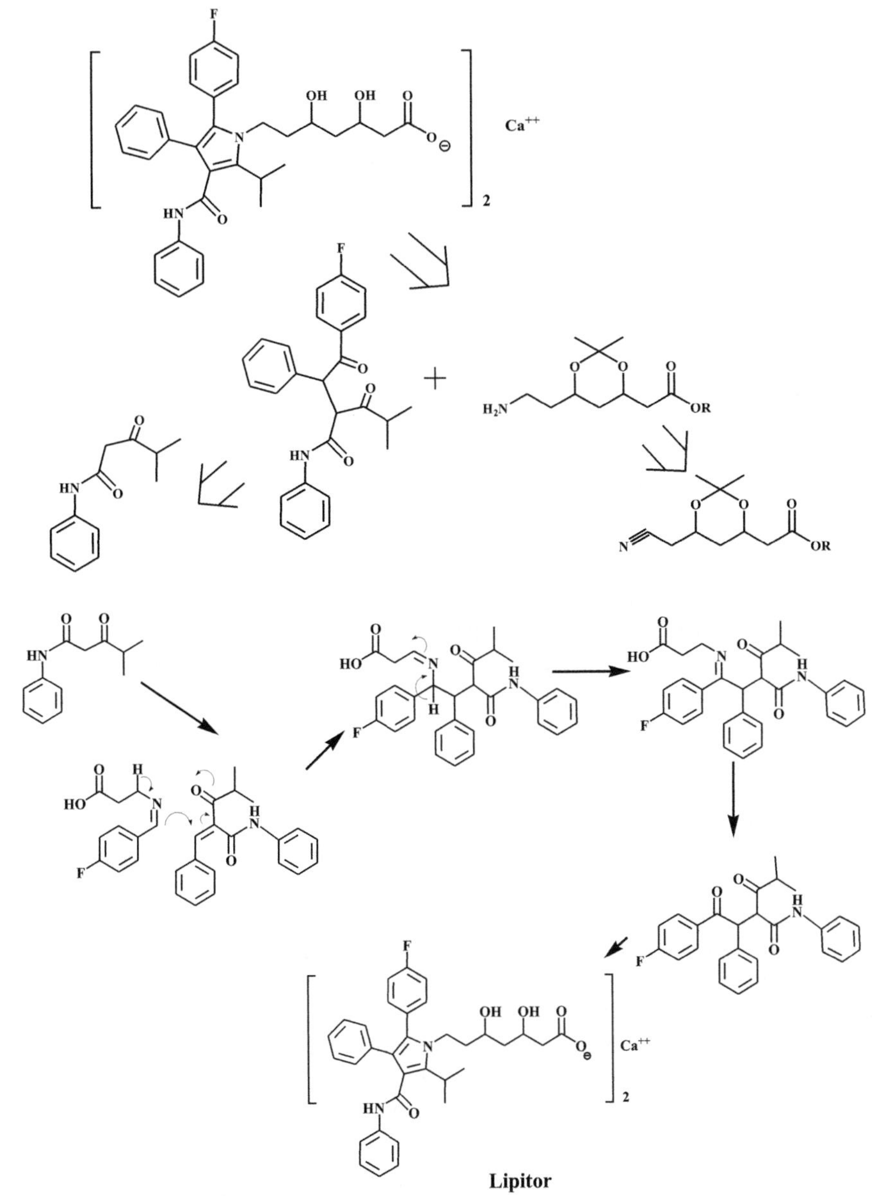

Lipitor

SCHEME 2.14 Retrosynthesis of Lipitor and synthesis of Lipitor.

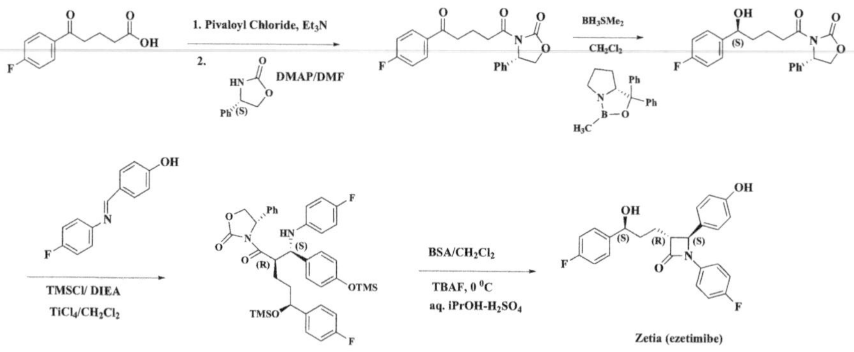

SCHEME 2.15   Synthesis of ezetimibe (Zetia).

2.5.2 Structure-Based Enzyme Inhibitors, e.g., HIV Protease Inhibitors

The discovery of HIV-1 protease inhibitors represents a classic example of structure-based drug design. Based on the knowledge of the x-ray crystal structure of HIV-1 protease, determined in 1989, many protease inhibitors were designed.[23] Two aspartic acid residues (Asp25 and Asp25'), present in the active site of the HIV-1 protease enzyme, are essential for the cleavage of the peptide bond. The protease inhibitors fit the active site of the HIV-1 aspartic protease and were designed to mimic the transition state of the proteases' natural substrate. The most promising transition state mimic was hydroxyethylamine, which led to the discovery of the first protease inhibitor, saquinavir. Using this principle other HIV-1 protease inhibitors were developed.

HIV-1 protease belongs to a family of aspartic acid proteases and exists as a homodimer of two 99 amino acid–containing proteins. The folding of the identical proteins leads to a C2 symmetric tertiary structure. Each monomer contributes an aspartic acid residue (Asp25 and Asp25′) that is essential for the hydrolysis of the scissile bond.

The HIV-1 protease inhibitors in clinical use have all the structural features necessary for tight binding into the active site of the enzyme. They are designed to include hydrophobic substituents that are clearly necessary for a tight fit in the hydrophobic binding pockets. Additionally, a feature common to nearly all the protease inhibitors is the presence of a free hydroxyl group, which plays an important role in hydrogen bonding directly with aspartic acid residues 25 and 25' in the active site. Another set of hydrogen bond acceptors allow hydrogen bonding to a conserved water molecule that is, in turn, hydrogen-bonded to isoleucine residues 50 and 50' of the protease backbone. Figure 2.19 illustrates these bindings with a pictorial representation of the drug, indinavir, as it fits into the active site of the HIV-1 protease.

HIV-1 protease inhibitors were considered a breakthrough in over a decade of AIDS research. Since HIV-1 protease inhibitors were first introduced in 1995, they have greatly benefited those infected by HIV-1 by suppressing the virus and reducing mortality. Examples of HIV-1 protease inhibitors approved by the FDA for clinical use are shown in Figures 2.20 and 2.21.

First-generation HIV-1 protease inhibitors were peptidomimetics, which displayed poor pharmacokinetics and gastrointestinal side effects and developed resistance. As

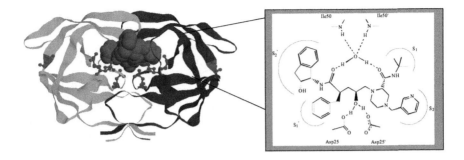

FIGURE 2.19   X-ray crystal structure of HIV-1 protease bound to the inhibitor (indinavir) (PDB code: 2avo).

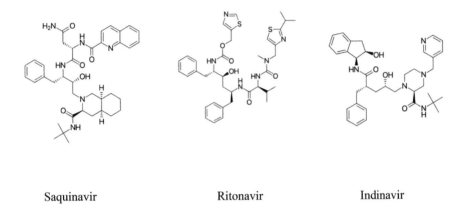

Saquinavir   Ritonavir   Indinavir

FIGURE 2.20   First-generation peptidomimetic HIV-1 protease inhibitors on the market.

the search for newer protease inhibitors continued, compounds containing a sulfonamide group as the binding moiety in place of an amide group were discovered, which improved the oral bioavailability. Subsequent modification of the end groups of these inhibitors resulted in stronger binding interactions with the protease backbone, resulting in enhanced activity against resistant organisms. Incorporation of end groups such as 3(S)-tetrahydrofuranyl urethane and bicyclic tetrahydrofuran (bis-THF) led to the discovery of the highly potent protease inhibitors amprenavir and darunavir (Figure 2.21).

All clinically available sulfonamide derived HIV-1 protease inhibitors, including amprenavir, tipranavir and darunavir, incorporate an open-chain, conformationally flexible sulfonamide group in their structures.[24] Based on the speculation that conformationally restricted cyclic sulfonamide HIV-1 protease inhibitors, represented by structure **1** (Figure 2.22)[25], might offer advantages over open-chain analogs by maximizing binding interactions with the backbone of the protease enzyme, several cyclic sulfonamides were synthesized. The general structure of cyclic sulfonamide represented by **1** offered an opportunity to explore biological activity associated with the lipophilicity and stereochemistry of the crucially important R' functionality.

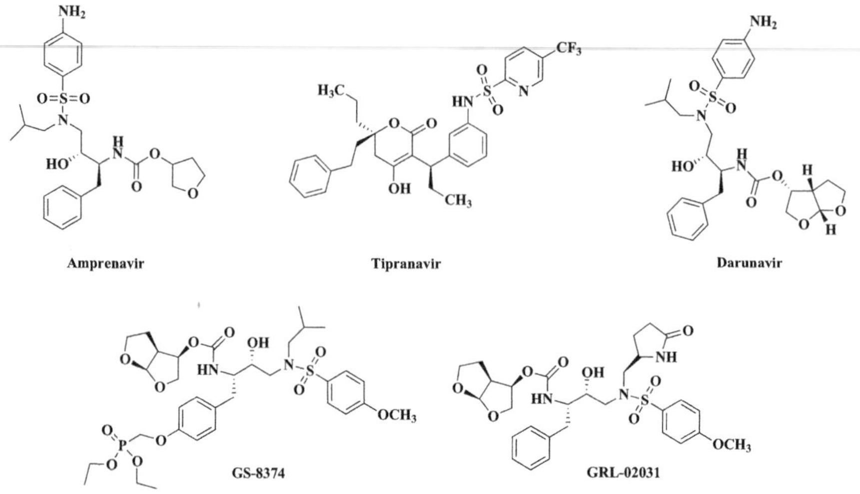

FIGURE 2.21   Protease inhibitors containing sulfonamide functional moiety.

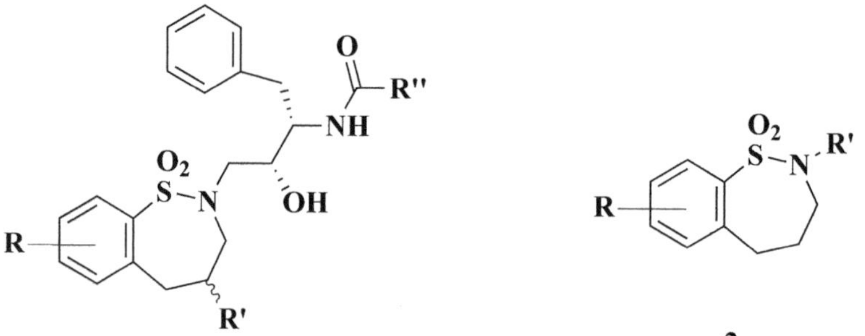

FIGURE 2.22   Design of novel cyclic sulfonamide HIV-1 protease inhibitors (core structure).

Compounds represented by structure **2** were synthesized using a radical cycliza-tion process.[26] Thus, treatment of compound **3** with tributyltin hydride (TBTH) and azobisisobutyronitrile (AIBN) in refluxing toluene solution yielded **2** via **4** and **5** (Scheme 2.16).

The aforementioned synthetic scheme has been extended to the synthesis of the cor-responding N-H compound **9** (Scheme 2.17). Treatment of 2-bromobenzenesulfonyl chloride (**6**) with allylamine (**7**) yielded the sulfonamide **8**. Radical reaction of **8** provided **9**. Treatment of **9** with the epoxide **10** furnished **11**. Compound **11** showed K_i of 470 nM in HIV-1 protease assay. Compound **11** was converted to compound **12** and found to be inactive, thus demonstrating the importance of the presence of the hydroxyl group and the carbamate in **11** for binding interactions.

Using a similar approach, compounds **9a–e** were synthesized from **8a–e**, respec-tively (Scheme 2.18).

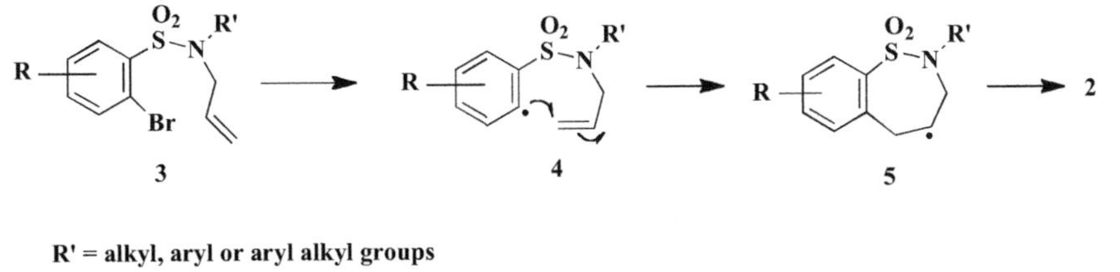

3
4
5
2
R' = alkyl, aryl or aryl alkyl groups

SCHEME 2.16 Synthesis of seven-membered cyclic sulfonamide using radical cyclization.

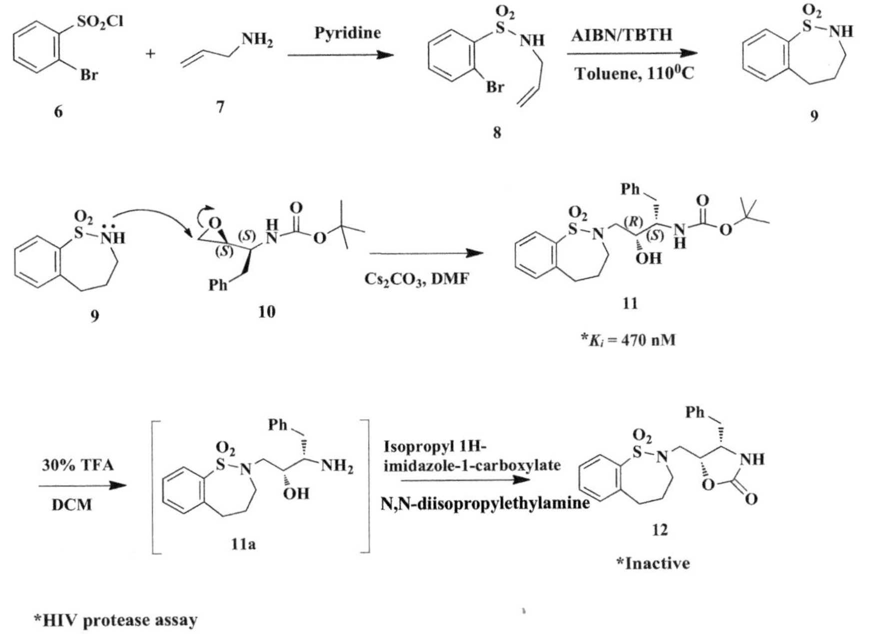

Pyridine
AIBN/TBTH
Toluene, 110°C
6
7
8
9
Cs2CO3, DMF
10
11
*Ki = 470 nM
30% TFA
DCM
11a
Isopropyl 1H-imidazole-1-carboxylate
N,N-diisopropylethylamine
12
*Inactive
*HIV protease assay

SCHEME 2.17 Synthesis of novel HIV-1 protease inhibitor **11**.

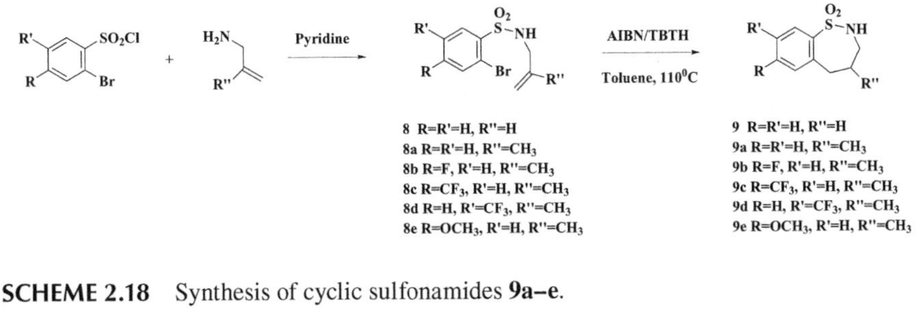

Pyridine
AIBN/TBTH
Toluene, 110°C
8 R=R'=H, R''=H
8a R=R'=H, R''=CH3
8b R=F, R'=H, R''=CH3
8c R=CF3, R'=H, R''=CH3
8d R=H, R'=CF3, R''=CH3
8e R=OCH3, R'=H, R''=CH3
9 R=R'=H, R''=H
9a R=R'=H, R''=CH3
9b R=F, R'=H, R''=CH3
9c R=CF3, R'=H, R''=CH3
9d R=H, R'=CF3, R''=CH3
9e R=OCH3, R'=H, R''=CH3

SCHEME 2.18 Synthesis of cyclic sulfonamides **9a–e**.

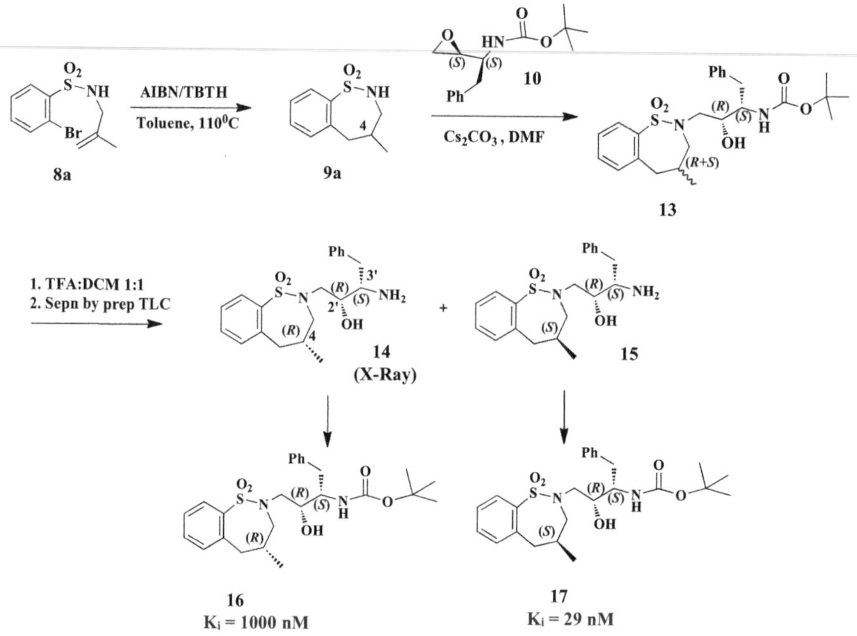

SCHEME 2.19 Synthesis of C4 methyl analogs.

Molecular modeling suggested that the introduction of a methyl group at C4 on the sulfonamide ring would enhance activity. Thus, radical cyclization of **8a** yielded racemate **9a**. Treatment of **9a** with the epoxide **10** yielded **13** as a mixture of diastereoisomers that could not be separated. Removal of the t-Boc group furnished the amine. At this stage the two diastereoisomers **14** and **15** could be separated. X-ray crystallographic analysis of **14** established its absolute stereochemistry as 4R, 2'R, 3'S (Figure 2.23), and therefore the absolute configuration of **15** would be 4S, 2'R, 3'S. Compounds **14** and **15** were then converted to the t-Boc derivatives **16** and **17**, respectively. In HIV-1 protease assay, **17** with K_i value of 29 nM was considerably more potent than **16**, which showed a K_i value of 1000 nm. This dramatic difference in protease inhibitory activity of **16** (4R,2'R,3'S) and **17** (4S,2'R,3'S) suggested the importance of the substituent and its stereochemistry at C4, which has to be (S) for optimum HIV-1 protease inhibitory activity. This demonstrated not only that the methyl group is important in improving potency but that it must also have the correct stereochemistry (Scheme 2.19).

For the next series of analogs, modifications at R1, R2, R3 led to synthesis of analogs **18–24** (Table 2.1). The C4(R) diastereoisomers, which are not shown here, were also analyzed in the protease assay and found to be inactive. Although **21** and **24** had nearly equal potency, it was preferred to advance **21** because it was likely to be more metabolically stable, as explained in the previous chapter.

The x-ray crystallographic structure of compound **21** bound to the HIV-1 protease (Figure 2.24)[25] showed that compound **21** occupied the active site cavity of the protease and made hydrogen bonding to the catalytic aspartic acid residues Asp25

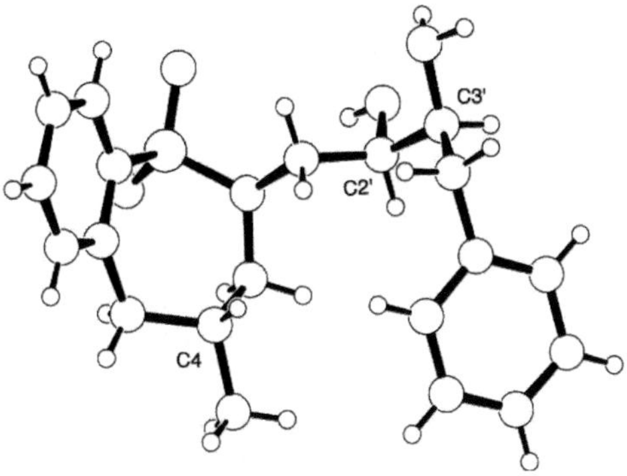

FIGURE 2.23 X-ray crystallographic structure of compound **14**.

TABLE 2.1

SAR of Novel HIV-1 Protease Inhibitors

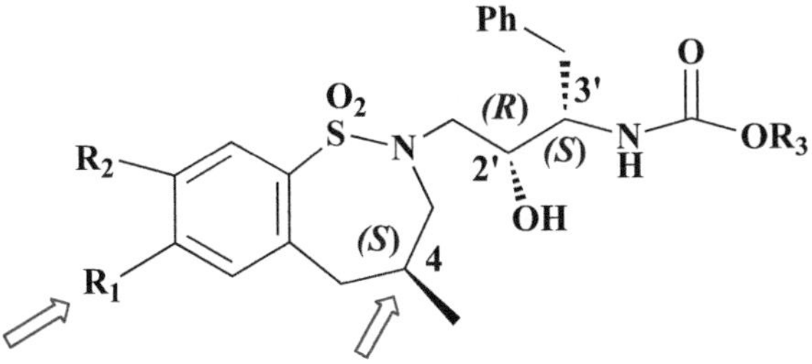

Compd No.	Substitution	K_i (nM)
18	$R_1=R_2=$ H; $R_3=$ Allyl	27
19	$R_1=R_2=$ H; $R_3=$ Et	34
20	$R_1=R_2=$ H; $R_3=$ Ph	350
21	$R_1=$ F; $R_2=$ H; $R_3=$ t-butyl	20
22	$R_1=$ CF$_3$; $R_2=$ H; $R_3=$ t-butyl	186
23	$R_1=$ H; $R_2=$ CF$_3$; $R_3=$ t-butyl	100
24	$R_1=$ OCH$_3$; $R_2=$ H; $R_3=$ t-butyl	19

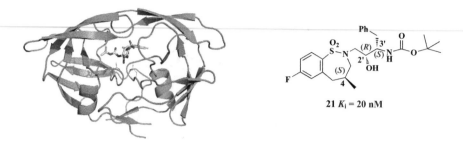

21 $K_i = 20$ nM

FIGURE 2.24 X-ray crystallographic structure of compound **21** bound to HIV-1 protease enzyme.

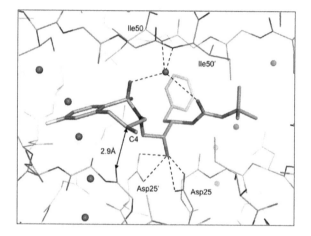

FIGURE 2.25 X-ray crystallographic structure of compound **21** showing key interactions with the HIV-1 protease enzyme.

and Asp25' through the hydroxyl group. The sulfonamide and carbamate carbonyl formed hydrogen bonds with a structural water molecule, which in turn hydrogen-bonded with Ile50 and Ile50' of the protease (Figure 2.25). In addition to these favorable hydrogen bonding stabilization effects, the C4-Me group of compound **21** has extensive hydrophobic interactions with the side chains of Leu23, Val82, and Ile84.

Furthermore, upon analyzing the x-ray crystallographic structure of compound **21** bound with HIV-1 protease, it was found that the C4-Me (S configuration) in compound **21** was 2.9 angstroms away from the carbonyl oxygen of Gly27' (Figure 2.26). If the C4-Me configuration was changed to (R) instead of (S), an unfavorable repulsion would be created between the C4-Me and the Gly27' carbonyl group and the interactions with the hydrophobic pocket would be lost. These results support the experimental observation that compounds with the C4 methyl group in the (S) configuration possess optimum activity.

The x-ray crystallographic analysis of compound **21** also suggested that the C4-Me group could be further extended to maximize the interactions with the hydrophobic

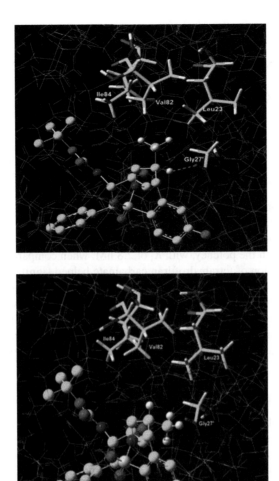

FIGURE 2.26 Molecular docking of compound **21** showing interactions of the C4(*S*) methyl group with the hydrophobic pocket and molecular docking of compound **21** with C4(*R*) methyl group showing no interactions with the hydrophobic pocket

pocket, thus enhancing potency. Hence, the effect of various alkyl groups at C4 on the cyclic sulfonamide ring with regard to their activity against HIV-1 protease was investigated. In addition, the molecular modeling suggested that tetrahydrofuran carbamates similar to amprenavir but different from darunavir would provide stronger binding to the protease backbone through hydrogen bonding of Asp29' and Asp30'. Thus, analogs represented by compound **25** and incorporating all the aforementioned ideas were synthesized (Figure 2.27).

Following multiple steps, the seven-membered cyclic sulfonamides with different R groups at C4 (Figure 2.27) were successfully prepared and converted into the

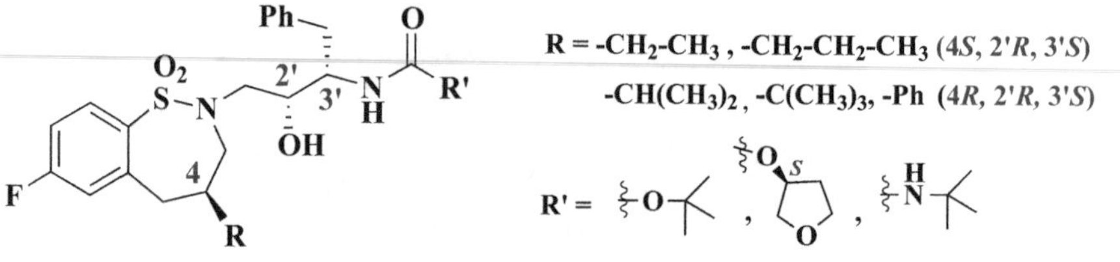

R = -CH$_2$-CH$_3$, -CH$_2$-CH$_2$-CH$_3$ (4S, 2'R, 3'S)

-CH(CH$_3$)$_2$, -C(CH$_3$)$_3$, -Ph (4R, 2'R, 3'S)

25

FIGURE 2.27   Design of novel analogs based on x-ray crystallographic analysis.

desired final products. The structures and their activities against HIV protease are shown in Table 2.2.

With the introduction of the C4-iPr (R) group in compound **28** there was a nearly six-fold increase in the potency, with K_i of 2.8 nM, when compared with compound **21**. The introduction of tetrahydrofuran carbamate helped significantly improve the activity in compound **29**, with a K_i of 360 pM. With a C4-t-butyl (R) group in compound **30**, there was further increase in activity when compared with compound **29**. Compound **30** was found to be the most potent analog, with a K_i of 260 pM.

The aforementioned detailed analysis is presented to demonstrate how the structure–activity relationship is established and the active analog identified for further development.

2.5.3 Substrate-based Enzyme Inhibitors, e.g., HCV Protease Inhibitors

The discovery of boceprevir, a drug used in the clinic for the treatment of HCV infection, was based on the concept of substrate-based drug design. The hepatitis C virus, or HCV, is an RNA virus that encodes a polypeptide that is post-translationally modified to mature virions. This process is carried out by a trypsin-like serine protease, thus resulting in the *cis* cleavage of the NS3-NS4A junction, followed by a *trans* cleavage of NS4A-NS4B, NS4B-NS5A, and NS5A-NS5B, thus producing a functional viral protein. Boceprevir from the Schering-Plough Research Institute and telaprevir from Vertex were discovered based on the concept of inhibiting the aforementioned serine protease, and they have been used in the clinic. However, better drugs have recently replaced them.

The starting point for the discovery of boceprevir[27] was the synthesis of compound **33** in which the scissile bond of the viral polypeptide was replaced by an α-ketoamide group, with the expectation that the ketone function would conjugate with the viral serine protease (Scheme 2.20). An identical sequence of the amino acid in the keto amide and the viral protein serves in the recognition process.

Although compound **33** was highly active (K_i = 0.0019 μM), its high molecular weight (MW) of 1265 suggested that it would not be a drug candidate. Lipinski's rule of five notes that most successful orally absorbable drugs have a molecular weight around 500. To achieve that goal, compound **33** had to be truncated on both the P and P' sites while maintaining activity. Thus, compound **34** was synthesized such that P2' to P5' were truncated. Compound **34** had a molecular weight of 796, which was

TABLE 2.2
Summary of Biological Activity in HIV-1 Protease Assay

Compound	Structure	K_i (nM)
Darunavir		<0.02
Amprenavir		0.08 ± 0.02
26		11 ± 1.1
27		28 ± 6
28		2.8 ± 1.9 3*
29		0.36 ± 0.1 0.43*
30		0.26 ± 0.05
31		34 ± 5.1
32		6.4 ± 1

*Replicate of HIV-1 assay at a different time

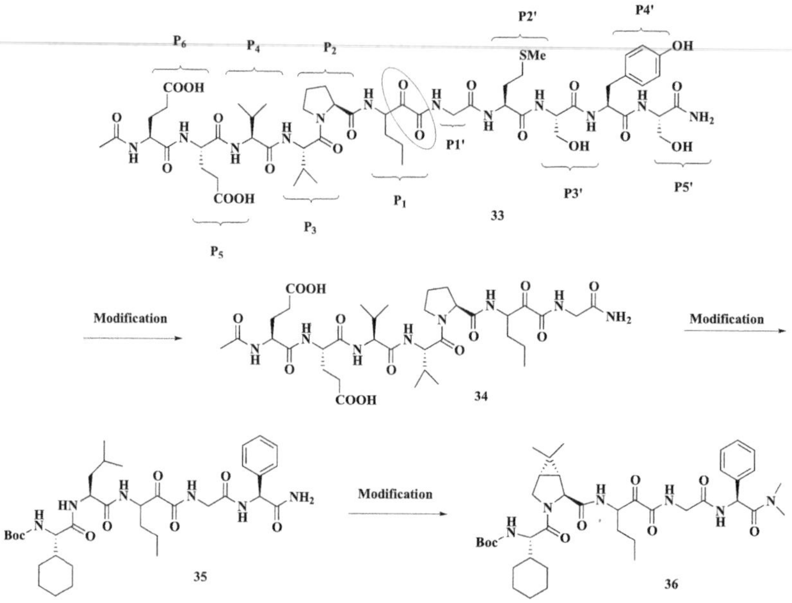

SCHEME 2.20 Initial lead modification for the discovery of boceprevir.

much lower than that of compound **33**, but it was also much less active (K_i = 0.043 µM). At this stage several analogs were designed, synthesized, and tested, leading to the identification of compounds **35** (K_i = 0.066 µM) and **36** (K_i = 0.01 µM), both of which were potent and possessed acceptable molecular weights. Although compound **36** was the most active thus far, it had poor bioavailability in various species of animals. To optimize bioavailability while maintaining potency, various changes were made in structure **36**, including incorporating different side chain residues at P1', P3, and P1 and capping the P3 site. These changes were guided by the availability of x-ray crystal structures of a few inhibitors bound to the NS3 protease. Thus, compound **37** (boceprevir, MW 519, K_i = 14 nM) was identified as the clinical candidate (Figure 2.28). It had a high degree of selectivity against related enzymes and acceptable oral bioavailability in various animal species. In rats it had a favorable distribution ratio of 30-fold in liver compared with plasma, which, if it translates to humans, will be of great clinical significance. The synthesis of boceprevir is presented in Scheme 2.21.

The x-ray crystal structure of **37** bound to the NS3 protease is shown in Figure 2.29.[27] The cyclobutyl alanine moiety occupied the S1 pocket and the dimethyl cyclopropyl proline residue in the bent conformation overlapped Ala156, His57, and Arg155. The side chain tertiary butyl glycine occupied the S3 pocket, the two of the methyl group in its structure interacted effectively with the protein, and the third was exposed to the solvent. The tertiary butyl urea group occupied the S4 pocket and the terminal NH₂ bonded to the protein backbone. With compound **37** locked into

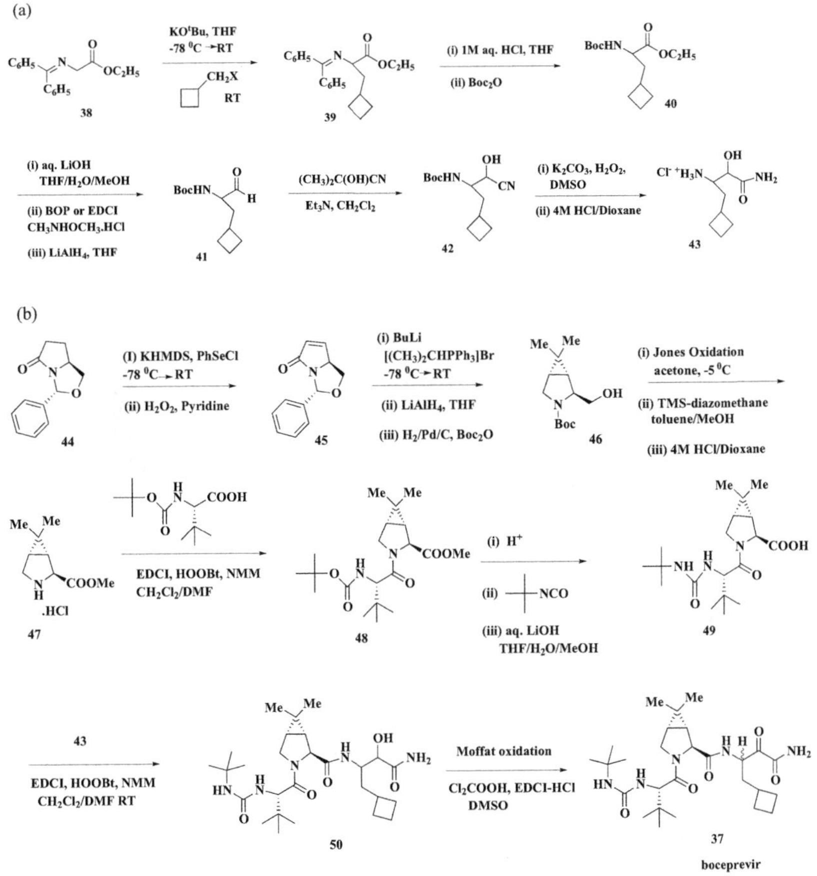

SCHEME 2.21   Synthesis of intermediate **43** and boceprevir.

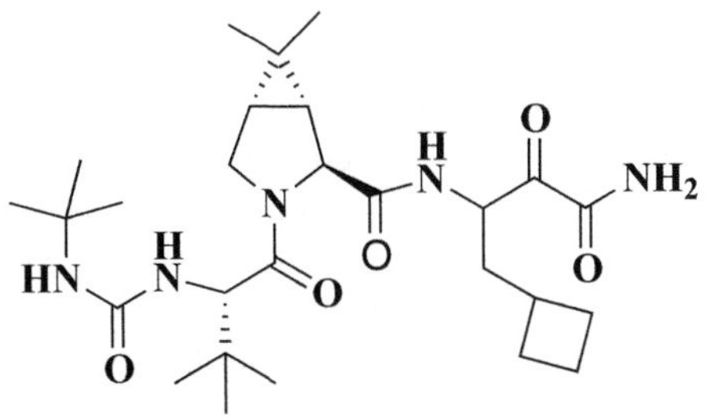

37

boceprevir

FIGURE 2.28   Structure of boceprevir (compound **37**).

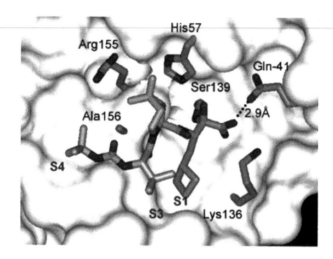

FIGURE 2.29   X-ray structure of boceprevir (**37**) bound to NS3 protease.

the protease pocket, Ser139 was now well positioned to reversibly bind covalently to the ketoamide, and the oxygen anion thus created was directed to the oxyanion hole.

2.5.4 MECHANISM-BASED ENZYME INHIBITORS, E.G., FPT INHIBITORS

The discovery of farnesyl protein transferase (FPT) inhibitors[28] represents an example of the mechanism-based approach to human cancer therapy. Ras proteins play a crucial role in many cellular signal transduction pathways, leading to cell activation and proliferation. The unregulated activity of Ras protein is implicated in nearly 30% of all human tumors. FPT catalyzes the attachment of the 15-carbon isoprenoid unit from farnesyl diphosphate (FPP) to the cysteine side chain of the conserved CAAX sequence (where C is cysteine; A is an aliphatic amino acid; and variable X is a methionine, serine, or alanine residue) located at the carboxy terminal of Ras. However, when X is leucine, the protein becomes geranylgeranylated, which uses the enzyme geranylgeranyl protein transferase (GGPT). The selectivity of FPT over GGPT is essential to avoid toxicity. Thus, selective FPT enzyme inhibition emerged as a promising approach for the treatment of cancer, which led to the discovery of lonafarnib (Sarasar), an orally active, selective nonpeptidic inhibitor.

Compound I, with a tricyclic ring system (IC_{50} = 250 nM), was identified by screening library of compounds, as an initial lead for the discovery of FPT inhibitors. Optimization of substitutions on rings A, B, C, D, and E in compound I was done using extensive chemical synthesis to bring the potency to the low-nanomolar range (Figure 2.30). Synthesis of 4-pyridylacetyl N-oxide of I (modification of E ring) showed greater FPT potency, with improved oral bioavailability and PK profile. Replacement of the 4-pyridylacetyl N-oxide moiety with a carboxamidopiperidin-ylacetyl group, as in compound III (IC_{50} = 49 nM), led to further improvement in potency, with excellent PK properties. The x-ray crystallographic structure of the

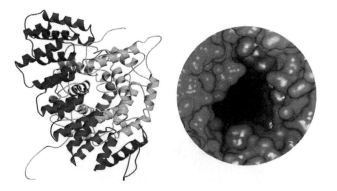

FIGURE 2.30   Structure of FPT inhibitors (initial lead compounds I, II, III, and lonafarnib).

FIGURE 2.31   X-ray crystal structure of FPT enzyme.

FPT enzyme shows a large active site cavity formed by the interaction of α and β subunits (Figure 2.31). Once the x-ray crystal structure[29] of the inhibitor bound to the enzyme is available, it is usually possible to design compounds, for example, by introducing lipophilic groups at appropriate centers in the molecule so that they will reach lipophilic sites in the structure of the protein, resulting in stronger binding, or by facilitating hydrogen bonding with the protein backbone either directly or with the use of an essential water molecule associated with the protein. Both of these ideas were incorporated into the structure of the inhibitor to optimize activity. Incorporation of the -CH$_2$ group to connect the amide group of ring D to E allowed hydrogen bonding of the inhibitor to the enzyme backbone with a structural water molecule, resulting in improved potency of the inhibitor by an order of magnitude. The S(-) enantiomer of the piperazine inhibitor (IIB) is more potent than the R(+) enantiomer (IIA), and their binding to the FPT enzyme is shown in Figure 2.32. Thus, strategically placed halogen atoms in rings A and C, guided by x-ray crystallographic analysis, resulted in analogs with stronger binding interactions with the FPT enzyme. Reduction of the double bond between rings B and D maintained activity while creating a new chiral center. The stereochemistry of the newly created chiral center in lonafarnib had a profound effect on FPT inhibitory activity. Among the trihalogenated tricyclic analogs, the R(+)isomer was found to be more potent than the

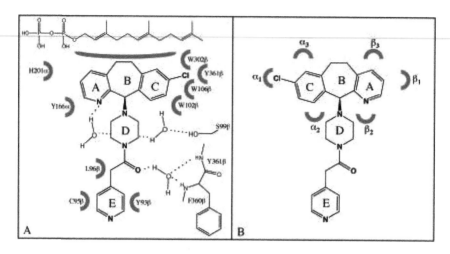

FIGURE 2.32 X-ray crystal structure of inhibitor IIA bound to FPT enzyme and inhibitor IIB bound to FPT enzyme.

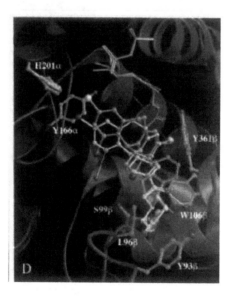

FIGURE 2.33 Overlay of the x-ray crystal structure of R(+) SCH 66336 (yellow) and S(-) SCH 66336 (purple) with the FPT enzyme.

S(-)isomer, which is due to the difference in binding mode between the two enantiomers (Figure 2.33). All of the aforementioned modifications led to the discovery of the selective, highly potent, orally active FPT inhibitor lonafarnib. It was advanced for clinical trials and found to be active against lung cancer; however, its activity in the clinic was not of sufficient interest to progress it further. More recently, lonafarnib was approved by the FDA for the treatment of progeria, a rare but devastating

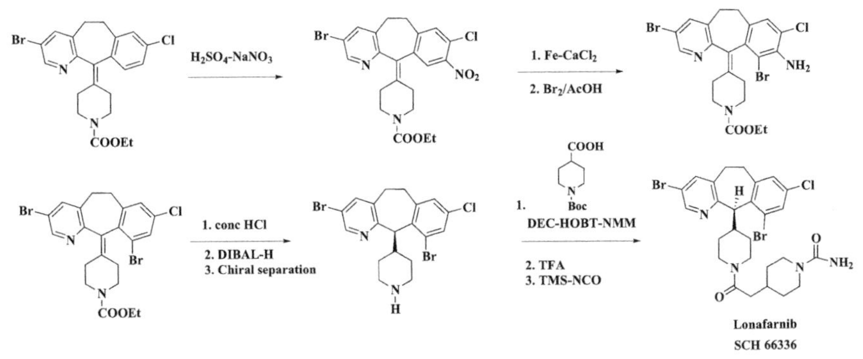

SCHEME 2.22   Synthesis of lonafarnib.

genetic disorder in children. Like Ras protein, progerin also gets farnesylated and causes progeria; therefore, Gordon[30] of Boston Children's Hospital argued for lonafarnib's use in the treatment of progeria.

The synthesis of lonafarnib[31] is shown in Scheme 2.22.

REFERENCES

1. Menard, R., and Storer, A. C. 1992. Oxyanion hole interactions in serine and cysteine proteases. *Biol. Chem. Hoppe-Seyler.* 373:393–400.
2. Robin, T., Reuveni, S., and Urbakh, M. 2018. Single-molecule theory of enzymatic inhibition. *Nat. Commun.* 9:779.
3. Jencks, W. P. 1987. *Catalysis in Chemistry and Enzymology,* Dover Publications Inc., New York, Chap. 1, 2, 3.
4. (a) Neitzel, J. J. 2010. Enzyme catalysis: The serine proteases. *Nature Education* 3(9):21. (b) Carter, P., and Wells, J. 1988. Dissecting the catalytic triad of a serine protease, Nature 332:564–568. (c) Blow, D., Birktoft, J., and Hartley, B. 1969. Role of a buried acid group in the mechanism of action of chymotrypsin. *Nature* 221:337–340. (d) Schoellman, G., and Shaw E. 1963. Direct evidence for the presence of histidine in the active center of chymotrypsin. *Biochemistry* 2:252–255.
5. Berg, J. M., Tymoczko, J. L., and Stryer, L. 2002. *Biochemistry,* 5th ed., W. H. Freeman, New York, Chap. 3.
6. Park, H. W., Boduluri, S. R., Moomaw, J. F., et al. 1997. Crystal structure of protein farnesyltransferase at 2.25 angstrom resolution. *Science* 275:1800–1804.
7. (a) Cushman, D., and Ondetti, M. A. 1999. Design of angiotensin converting enzyme inhibitors. *Nat. Med.* 5:1110–1112. (b) Cushman, D. W., and Ondetti, M. A. 1991. History of the design of captopril and related inhibitors of angiotensin converting enzyme. *Hypertension* 17(4):589–592. (c) Davis, S. 2007. Enalapril. In *xPharm: The Comprehensive Pharmacology Reference*, Elsevier, New York, pp. 1–6.
8. (a) Tobert J. A. 2003. Lovastatin and beyond: The history of the HMG-CoA reductase inhibitors. *Nat. Rev. Drug Discov.* 2(7):517–526. (b) Hartman G. D., Halczenko, W., Duggan, M. E., et al. 1992. 3-Hydroxy-3-methylglutaryl-coenzyme A reductase inhibitors. 9. The synthesis and biological evaluation of novel simvastatin analogs. *J. Med. Chem.* 35(21):3813–3821. (c) Baumann, K. L., Butler, D. E., Deering, C. F., et al. 1992. The convergent synthesis of CI-981, an optically active, highly potent, tissue selective inhibitor of HMG-CoA reductase. *Tetrahedron Lett.* 33(17):2283–2284.

9. Mainwright, M., and Kristiansen, J. E. 2011. On the 75th anniversary of Prontosil. *Dyes and Pigments.* 88(3):231–234.

10. (a) Woods, D. D. 1940. The relation of p-aminobenzoic acid to the mechanism of the action of sulphanilamide. *Brit. J. Exp. Pathol.* 21:74–90. (b) Hitchings G. H. 1973. Mechanism of action of trimethoprim-sulfamethoxazole. I. *J. Infect. Dis.* 128:433–436.

11. (a) Fleming, A. 1929. On the antibacterial action of cultures of a Pencillium, with special reference to their use in the isolation of *B. influenzae. Br. J. Exp. Pathol.* 10:226–236. (b) Wainwright, M. 1990. *Miracle Cure: The Story of Penicillin and the Golden Age of Antibiotics,* Basil Blackwell, Oxford, 38–48.

12. Blumberg, P. M., and J. L. Strominger. 1974. Interaction of penicillin with the bacterial cell: Penicillin-binding proteins and penicillin-sensitive enzymes. *Bacteriol. Rev.* 38:291–335. (b) Barbour, A. G. 1981. Properties of penicillin-binding proteins in Neisseria gonorrhoeae. *Antimicrob. Agents Chemother.* 19:316–322.

13. Yotsuji, A., Mitsuyama, J., Hori, R., et al. 1988. Mechanism of action of cephalosporins and resistance caused by decreased affinity for penicillin-binding proteins in *Bacteroides fragilis. Antimicrob. Agents and Chemother.* 32:1848–1853.

14. (a) Baldwin, J. E., and Abraham E. 1988. The biosynthesis of penicillins and cephalosporins. *Nat. Prod. Rep.* 5(2):129–145. (b) Demain, A. L. 1966. Biosynthesis of penicillins and cephalosporins. In *Biosynthesis of Antibiotics.* Ed. Snell, J. F. Academic Press Inc., New York, Chap. 2.

15. (a) Morin, R. B., Jackson, B. G., Mueller, R. A., et al. 1963. Chemistry of cephalosporin antibiotics. III. Chemical correlation of penicillin and cephalosporin antibiotics. *J. Amer. Chem. Soc.* 85(12):1896–1897. (b) Morin, R. B., Jackson, B. G., and Mueller, R. A. 1969. Chemistry of cephalosporin antibiotics. XV. Transformations of penicillin sulfoxide. Synthesis of cephalosporin compounds. *J. Amer. Chem. Soc.* 91:1401–1407. (c) Spry. D. O. 1970. Conversion of penicillin to cephalosporin via a double sulfoxide rearrangement. *J. Am. Chem. Soc.* 92(16):5006–5008.

16. (a) Jelic, D., and Antolovic, R. 2016. From erythromycin to azithromycin and new potential ribosome-binding antimicrobials. *Antibiotics* 5:29. (b) Lee, Y., Choi, J. Y., Fu, H., et al. 2011. Chemistry and biology of macrolide antiparasitic agents. *J. Med. Chem.* 54:2792–2804.

17. Sheehan, D, J., Hitchcock, C. A., and Sibley, C. M. 1999. Current and emerging azole antifungal agents. *Clin. Microb. Rev.* 12(1):40–79.

18. (a) Saksena, A. K., Girijavallabhan, V. M., Lovery, R. G., et al. 1995. SCH 51048, A novel broad-spectrum orally active antifungal agent: Synthesis and preliminary structure-activity profile. *Biorg. Med. Chem. Lett.* 5(2):127–132. (b) Saksena, A. K., Girijavallabhan, V. M., Wang, H., et al. 1996. Concise asymmetric routes to 2,2,4-trisubstituted tetrahydrofurans via chiral titanium imide enolates: Key intermediates towards synthesis of highly active azole antifungals SCH 51048 AND SCH 56592. *Tetrahedron Lett.* 37(32):5657–5660.

19. Bennett, F., Saksena, A. K., Lovey, R. G., et al. 2006. Hydroxylated analogues of the orally active broad spectrum antifungal, Sch 51048(1), and the discovery of posaconazole [Sch 56592; 2 or (S,S)-5]. *Bioorg. Med. Chem. Lett.* 16:186–190.

20. Cerqueira, N. M. F. S. A., Eduardo F., Oliveira, D. S., et al. 2016. Cholesterol Biosynthesis: A Mechanistic Overview. *Biochemistry* 55:5483–5506.

21. Baumann, K. L., Butler, D. E., and Deering, C. F., et al. 1992. The convergent synthesis of CI-981, an optically active, highly potent, tissue selective inhibitor of HMG-CoA reductase. *Tetrahedron Lett.* 33(17):2283–2284.

22. Clader, J. W. 2004. The discovery of Ezetimibe: A view from outside the receptor. *J. Med. chem.* 47(1):1–9.

23. Wlodawer, A., and Vondrasek, J. 1998. Inhibitors of HIV-1 protease: A major success of structure assisted drug design. *Annu. Rev. Biophys. Biomol. Struct.* 2:249–284.

24. (a) Raza, A., Sham, Y., and Vince, R. 2008. Design and synthesis of sulfoximine based inhibitors for HIV-1 protease. *Bioorg. Med. Chem. Lett.* 18:5406–5410. (b) Koh, Y., Nakata, H., Maeda, K., et al. 2003. Novel bis-tetrahydro furanylurethane containing non-peptidic protease inhibitor (PI) UIC-94017 (TMC114) with potent activity against multi-PI-resistant human immunodeficiency virus invitro. *Antimicrob. Agents Chemother.* 47:3123–3129.

25. (a) Ganguly, A. K., Alluri, S. S., Caroccia, D., et al. 2011. Design, synthesis and x-ray crystallographic analysis of a novel class of HIV-1 protease inhibitors. *J. Med. Chem.* 54:7176–7183. (b) Ganguly, A. K., Alluri, S. S., Wang C-H., et al. 2014. Structural optimization of cyclic sulfonamide based novel HIV-1 protease inhibitors to picomolar affinities guided by x-ray crystallographic analysis. *Tetrahedron* 70:2894–2904. (c) Alluri, S. S., and Ganguly, A. K. 2018. Design and synthesis of HIV-1 protease inhibitors. *Frontiers in Clinical Drug Research-HIV* 4:1–33.

26. Biswas, D., Samp, L., and Ganguly, A. K. 2010. Synthesis of conformationally restricted sulfonamides via radical cyclisation. *Tetrahedron Lett.* 51:2681–2684.

27. Venkatraman, S., Bogen, S. L., Arasappan, A., et al. 2006. Discovery of (1R,5S)-N-[3-Amino-1-(cyclobutylmethyl)-2,3-dioxopropyl]-3-[2(S)-[[[(1,1-dimethylethyl)amino] carbonyl]amino]-3,3-dimethyl-1-oxobutyl]-6,6-dimethyl-3-azabicyclo[3.1.0]hexan-2(S)-carboxamide (SCH 503034), a selective, potent, orally bioavailable hepatitis C virus NS3 protease inhibitor: A potential therapeutic agent for the treatment of hepatitis C infection. *J. Med. Chem.* 49:6074–6086.

28. Njorge, F. G., Doll, R. J., Vibulbhan, B., et al. 1997. Discovery of non-peptide tricyclic inhibitors of Ras farnesyl protein transferase. *Biorg. Med. Chem.* 5(1):101–113.

29. Strickland, C. L., Weber, P. C., Windsor, W. T., et al. 1999. Tricyclic farnesyl protein transferase inhibitors: Crystallographic and calorimetric studies of structure-activity relationships. *J. Med. Chem.* 42:2125–2135.

30. Gordon, L. B., Kleinman, M. E., Miller, D. T. 2012. Clinical trial of a farnesyltransferase inhibitor in children with Hutchinson-Gilford progeria syndrome. *PNAS* 109(41):16666–16671.

31. (a) Ganguly, A. K., Doll, R. J., and Girijavallabhan, V. M. 2001. Farnesyl protein transferase inhibition: A novel approach to antitumor therapy. The discovery and development of SCH66336. *Curr. Med. Chem.* 8:1419–1436. (b) Njorge, G. F., Taveras, A. G., Kelly, J., et al. 1998. (+)-4-[2-[4-(8-Chloro-3,10-dibromo-6,11-dihydro-5H-benzo[5,6] cyclohepta[1,2-b]-pyridin-11(R)-yl]-1-piperidinyl]-2-oxo-ethyl]-1-piperidinecarboxamid e(SCH-66336): A very potent farnesyl protein transferase inhibitor as a novel antitumor agent. *J. Med. Chem.* 41:4890–4902.

3 Receptor Agonists and Antagonists

Pharmacokinetics involve the study of the absorption, distribution, metabolism, and excretion (ADME) of a drug substance. Pharmacodynamics is the study of the interaction of the drug with its targets, including receptors and enzymes (sites of action). Receptors[1] are polypeptide macromolecules that can be membrane-bound, such as the G protein-coupled receptors (GPCRs),[2] and function in a membrane environment containing cholesterol and phosphatidylcholine or inside cells as intracellular receptors, such as nuclear receptors (Figure 3.1). Cell membranes perform the essential function of protecting the cell from water-soluble substances and providing a surface to which enzymes and proteins can attach to provide localization and structural organization. As many receptors are membrane-bound, very often they cannot be crystallized, and hence structural information based on x-ray analysis of receptors is rarely available. Therefore, characterizations of receptors are based on their function.

The biological activity of a drug is related to its affinity to the receptor, which is measured as a dissociation constant (K_D). A smaller K_D indicates higher affinity of the drug to the receptor (i.e., greater activity).

$$\text{Drug} + \text{Receptor} \underset{k_{off}}{\overset{k_{on}}{\rightleftharpoons}} \text{Drug–receptor complex}$$

$$K_d = \frac{[\text{Drug}][\text{Receptor}]}{[\text{Drug–receptor complex}]}$$

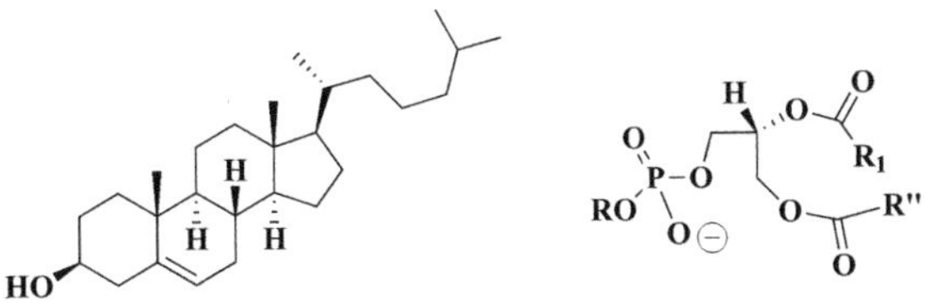

$R = CH_2CH_2N(CH_3)_3^+$
$R',R'' = \text{long hydrocarbon chains}$

Cholesterol   Phosphatidylcholine

FIGURE 3.1 Drug–receptor interaction and dissociation constant and structure of cholesterol and phosphatidylcholine.

DOI: 10.1201/9781003182573-3

3.1 AGONIST AND ANTAGONIST

The binding of a drug or natural ligand to the receptor results in various cellular responses, as described next. Agonists elicit biological activity when they occupy receptors (e.g., hormones, neurotransmitters). The rates of association and dissociation of agonists are fast. An antagonist binds to receptors but does not activate them. It neutralizes the activity associated with the agonist. The rate of association of antagonists will be fast, and the rate of dissociation will be slow. A competitive antagonist by itself does not produce any activity; however, when added in increasing amounts to an agonist, the agonist's activity is diminished. Therefore, both the agonist and the antagonist bind to the same site of the receptor. A noncompetitive antagonist binds to an allosteric site of the receptor and reduces the magnitude of the maximum response of the agonist dose–response curve.

Acetylcholine causes muscle contractions (CNS-mediated) by binding to its receptor; when an agonist is added, the curve does not change. However, when an antagonist is added, muscle contractions associated with acetylcholine are neutralized. This also implies that acetylcholine and the agonist bind to the same site of the receptor (Figure 3.2).

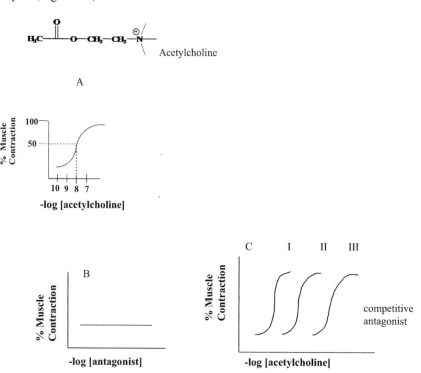

FIGURE 3.2   Dose response curve for (A) full agonist; (B) antagonist; (C) I, no antagonist present; II, III, with increasing concentrations of antagonist.

3.2 FACTORS INVOLVED IN THE FORMATION OF A DRUG–RECEPTOR COMPLEX

3.2.1 HYDROGEN BONDS

Hydrogen bonds occur both inter- and intramolecularly as long as the hydrogen bonding element is within approximately 1.9 Å (Figure 3.3).

3.2.2 ELECTROSTATIC FORCES

At physiological pH basic amine groups of lysine, arginine, and histidine are protonated and acidic carboxylic groups of aspartic acid and glutamic acid are deprotonated. The attractive interactions between the oppositely charged groups will aid in drug–receptor binding (Figure 3.4).

3.2.3 CHARGE–TRANSFER COMPLEXES

When two molecules, one of which is an electron donor and one of which is an electron acceptor, come into contact, they form a charge–transfer complex (Figure 3.5).

3.2.4 VAN DER WAALS FORCES

Weak forces occur when molecules or a group of atoms are in close contact with another (~ 4Å). When atoms are too close to each other the electron clouds repel each other. The balance of attractive and repulsive forces leads to an optimum distance

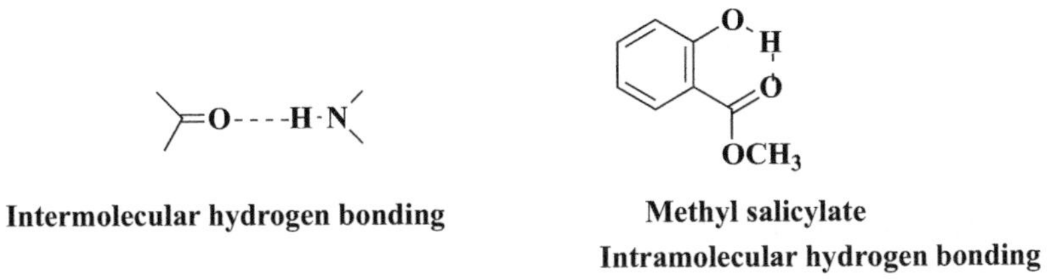

Intermolecular hydrogen bonding

Methyl salicylate
Intramolecular hydrogen bonding

FIGURE 3.3   Hydrogen bonding in molecules.

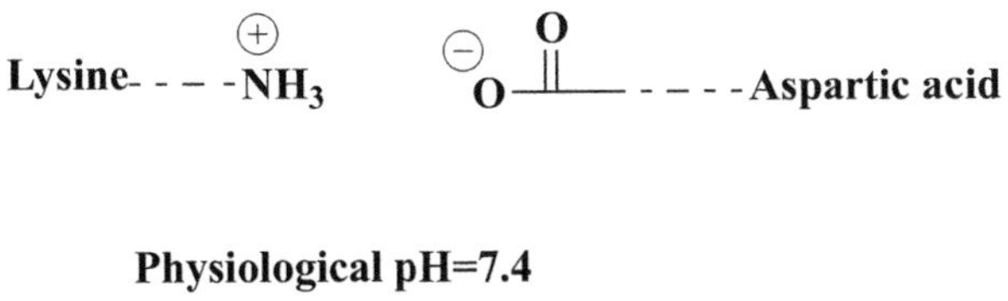

Lysine- - - -$\overset{\oplus}{N}H_3$ $\overset{\ominus}{O}$—$\overset{O}{\overset{\|}{}}$- - - - - Aspartic acid

Physiological pH=7.4

FIGURE 3.4   Electrostatic interactions between amino and carboxylic groups.

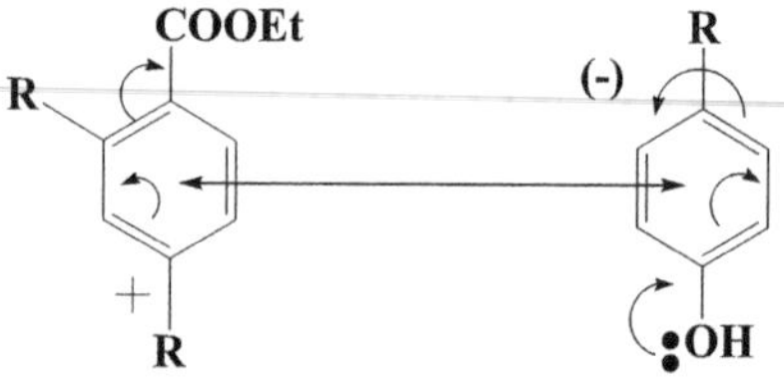

FIGURE 3.5. Formation of a charge–transfer complex.

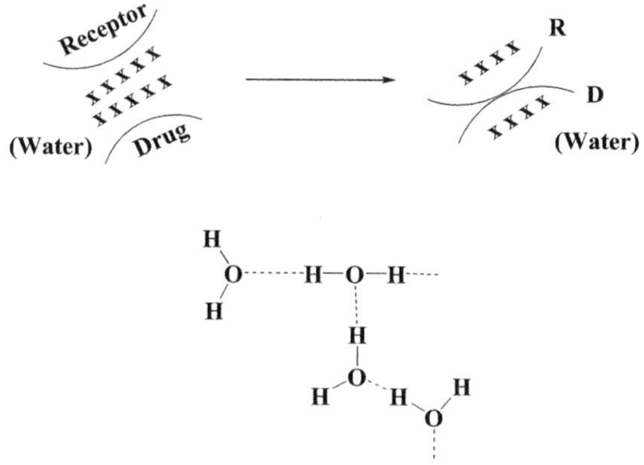

FIGURE 3.6 Hydrophobic interactions between receptor and drug.

(i.e., the van der Waals distance) between the atoms. This is the sum of the van der Waals radii of the atoms concerned. Van der Waals interactions are weaker interactions than hydrogen bonds, and they can become significant when two nonpolar molecular surfaces are complementary in shape and size.

3.2.5 HYDROPHOBIC FORCES

Hydrophobic groups associate with each other and remain buried in the protein tertiary structures and away from water molecules. Thus, when the lipophilic drug molecule and nonpolar receptor group approach each other, the water molecules between them become disordered in an attempt to associate with each other, resulting in a drug–receptor complex (Figure 3.6).

3.3 DRUG–RECEPTOR CHIRALITY

As receptors are macromolecular polypeptides, they are chiral. In a chiral drug[4] it is usually one enantiomer that is active because it is recognized by chiral receptors. Enantiomers can have different activities; for example, in the case of thalidomide, one enantiomer is active and the other is toxic. A couple more examples of this phenomenon are shown in Figure 3.7. It should be noted that a drug does not have to

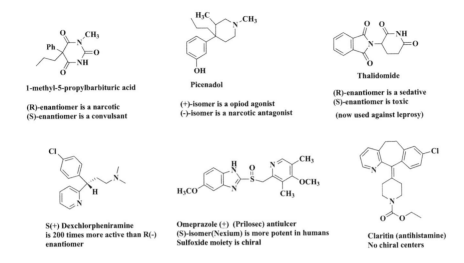

FIGURE 3.7 Examples of chiral and achiral drugs.

be chiral to bind to a receptor; for example, Claritin is achiral and is a very potent histamine H1 receptor antagonist.

3.4 HISTAMINE RECEPTORS

Histamine[5,6] is a potent bronchoconstrictive agent, and when released it initiates an allergic response. There are three subclasses of histamine receptors (i.e., H1, H2, and H3), and when they are occupied by histamine, they elicit different biological responses (Figure 3.8). For example, occupation of the histamine H1 receptor causes allergic responses and occupation of the histamine H2 receptor causes ulcers.

3.4.1 H1 Receptor Antagonists

The general structural features of more commonly used H1-antihistamines are shown in Figure 3.9.

Azatadine is a potent first-generation H1 receptor antagonist in clinical use (Figure 3.10). It shows inhibition of histamine-induced contraction of guinea pig ileum (IC_{50} = 2.5 nM) and activity in response to histamine-induced lethality in guinea pigs (ED_{50} = 0.009 mg/kg p.o.). However, azatadine was found to have CNS activity (electroconvulsive seizures: ED_{50} >80 mg/kg p.o.; acetic acid–induced writh-ing: ED_{50} = 8.9 mg/kg p.o.; physostigmine lethality: ED_{50} = 6.1 mg/kg p.o.) in mice, indicating its sedating effect.

With the goal of developing a potent H1-antihistamine with nonsedative proper-ties, several structural modifications on the aromatic and piperidine ring of azatadine were made, which led to the discovery of Claritin (loratadine).[7,8] The basic nitrogen of the piperidine ring was converted to amides, sulfonamides, urea, and carbamates. An ethyl carbamate substitution (Figure 3.10) on the nitrogen resulted in the most potent

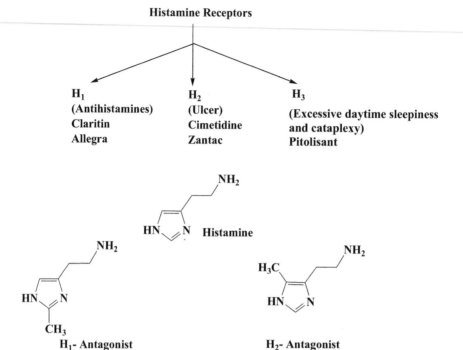

FIGURE 3.8 Types of histamine receptors and their antagonists.

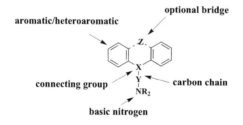

FIGURE 3.9 H1-antihistamine structural features.

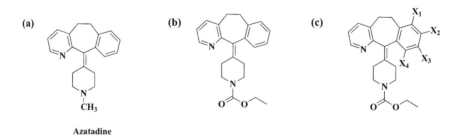

FIGURE 3.10 (a) structure of azatadine (b) substitution on the piperidine nitrogen (c) substitution on the aromatic ring.

compound (histamine-induced lethality in guinea pigs: $ED_{50} = 0.79$ mg/kg p.o.) and also showed higher ED_{50} in the CNS activity (electroconvulsive seizures: $ED_{50} >$ 320 mg/kg p.o.; acetic acid–induced writhing: $ED_{50} = 160$ mg/kg p.o.; physostigmine lethality: $ED_{50} > 160$ mg/kg p.o. in mice), indicating less potential to cause sedation. Adding an ethyl carbamate yielded a compound with good efficacy and safety; however, the compound had a short half-life. To solve this problem, several compounds were made by substituting the aromatic ring with a halogen group in an effort to block the aromatic ring metabolism. The compound with chlorine at X_2 was found to be the most potent in this series (histamine induced lethality in guinea pigs $ED_{50} =$ 0.19 mg/kg p.o.) and showed a long half-life and did not produce sedation (electroconvulsive seizures: $ED_{50} > 320$ mg/kg p.o.; acetic acid–induced writhing: $ED_{50} >$ 320 mg/kg p.o.; physostigmine lethality: $ED_{50} > 320$ mg/kg p.o. in mice). Thus, this compound, known as Claritin, became the first nonsedative antihistamine.

Claritin and Allegra are widely used in the clinic as nonsedative antihistamines (Figure 3.11). The synthesis of Claritin is shown in Scheme 3.1. Allegra[9] is a

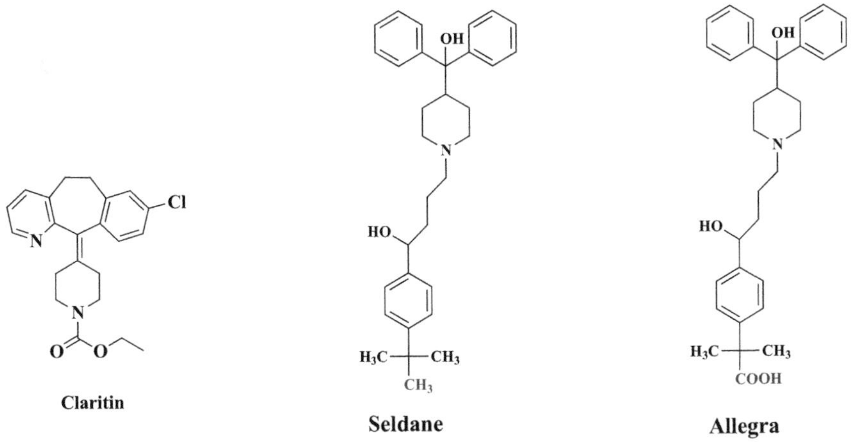

FIGURE 3.11   Structure of Claritin, Seldane, and Allegra.

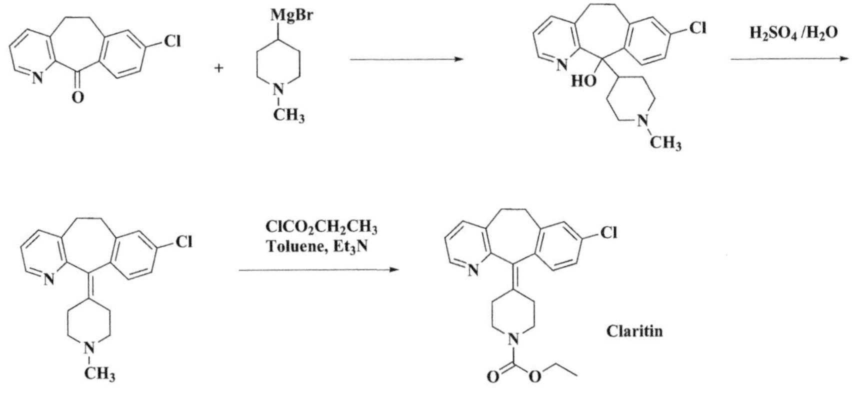

SCHEME 3.1   Synthesis of Claritin.

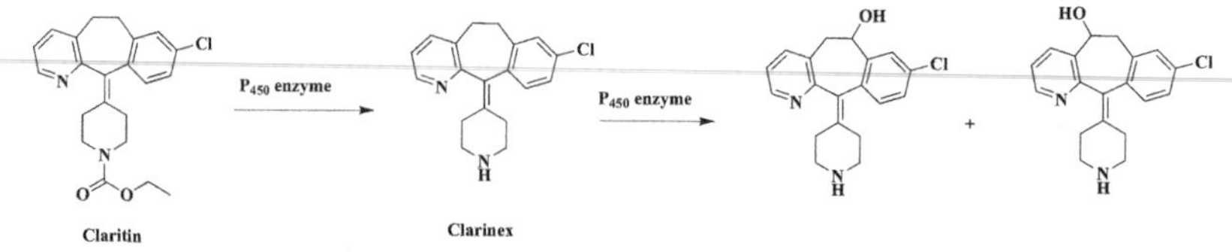

FIGURE 3.12   Metabolites of Claritin.

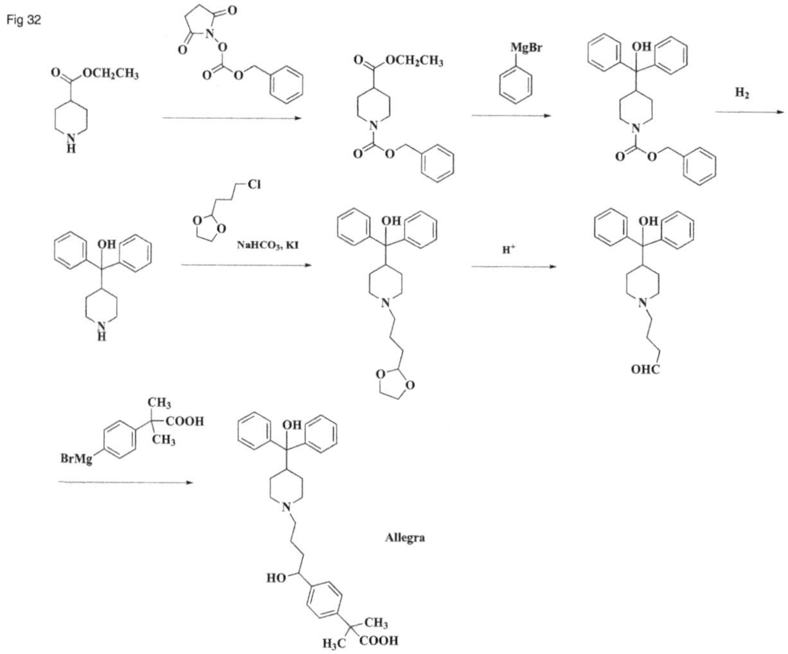

SCHEME 3.2   Synthesis of Allegra.

metabolite of Seldane and was observed when Seldane was administered to humans. It did not show the cardiac arrhythmia side effects associated with Seldane.

The structures of various metabolites of Claritin are shown in Figure 3.12. Clarinex, the major metabolite of Claritin, is clinically used for the treatment of allergic rhinitis.

The synthesis of Allegra is shown in Scheme 3.2.

3.4.2 H2 Receptor Antagonists

Histamine bound to H2 receptors in the stomach leads to the release of acid, which causes gastric ulcers. H2 receptor antagonists are therefore useful in the treatment of ulcers. The progression toward the discovery of cimetidine,[10] the first example of an orally active antiulcer agent, is outlined in Figure 3.13 and Scheme 3.3.

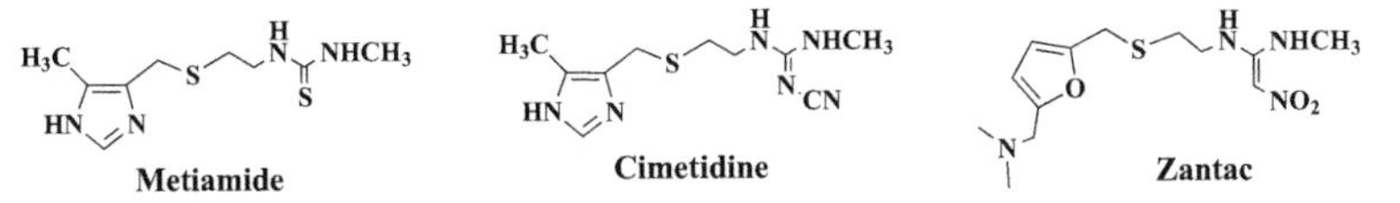

FIGURE 3.13 Structure of metiamide, cimetidine, and ranitidine (Zantac).

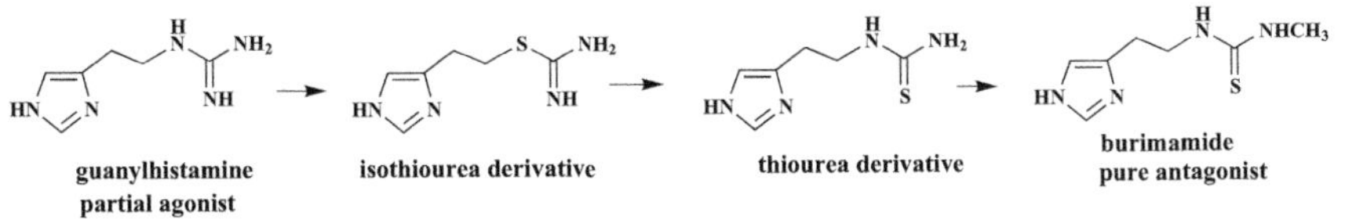

SCHEME 3.3 Discovery of H2 receptor antagonists.

The discovery of cimetidine began with the synthesis of guanylhistamine, which exhibited partial agonistic activity by mimicking the action of histamine and triggering acid release in the stomach (Scheme 3.3). Isosteric replacement of a nitrogen with sulfur yielded the isothiourea derivative, which provided enhanced potency as an H2 antagonist. It was realized that if the side chain acquired an electronic property, as in the case of histamine, acid-releasing activity would remain. This was avoided by incorporating a thiourea group, and subsequent derivatization led to the synthesis of burimamide, which was a pure antagonist; however, it showed no oral absorption in humans.

By careful consideration of electronic effects influencing the disposition of the hydrogen atoms in the imidazole ring, metiamide was synthesized and found to be ten times more potent than burimamide and orally active. However, there were side effects associated with metiamide attributable to the presence of the thiourea group. By replacing the thiourea group in metiamide with a different polar group, cimetidine was synthesized and found to be a potent, orally active H2 receptor antagonist. It competitively inhibited the binding of histamine to H2 receptors and had almost no effect on H1 receptors. Cimetidine has a half-life of only 2 hours and was succeeded by the longer acting and more potent H2 receptor antagonist ranitidine (Zantac). However, ranitidine has recently been withdrawn from the market because commercial batches were found to be contaminated with N-nitrosodimethylamine (NDMA), a human carcinogen (Figure 3.13).

The synthesis of cimetidine is shown in Scheme 3.4.

Replacing the imidazole ring in cimetidine with its surrogate resulted in the discovery of the more potent drug ranitidine (Zantac).[11] Interactions of Zantac with the receptor are shown in Figure 3.14, and its synthesis is presented in Scheme 3.5.

3.5 ANGIOTENSIN II RECEPTOR ANTAGONISTS

The renin-angiotensin-aldosterone (RAS) system plays a key role in regulating blood pressure in humans. High blood pressure is caused by a sequence of events, starting from the release of a protein, angiotensinogen, in the liver. Renin cleaves

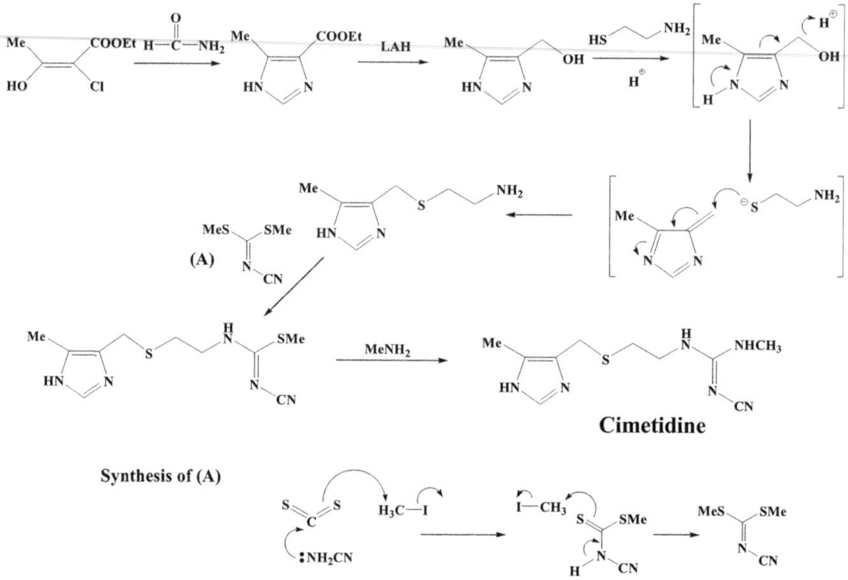

SCHEME 3.4 Synthesis of cimetidine.

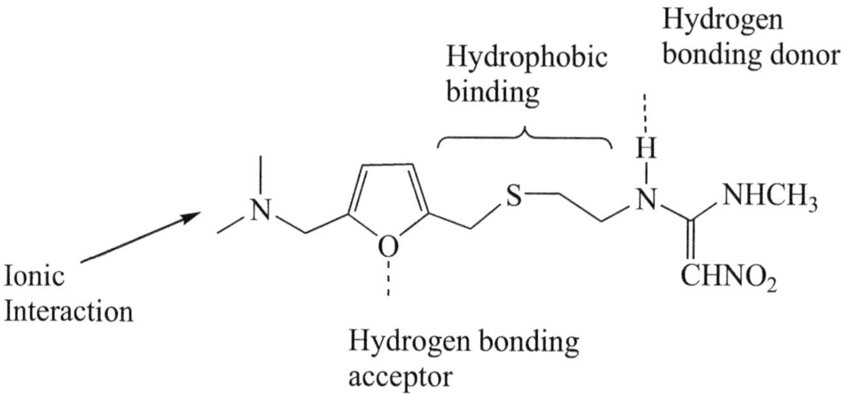

FIGURE 3.14 Interactions of Zantac with histamine H2 receptor.

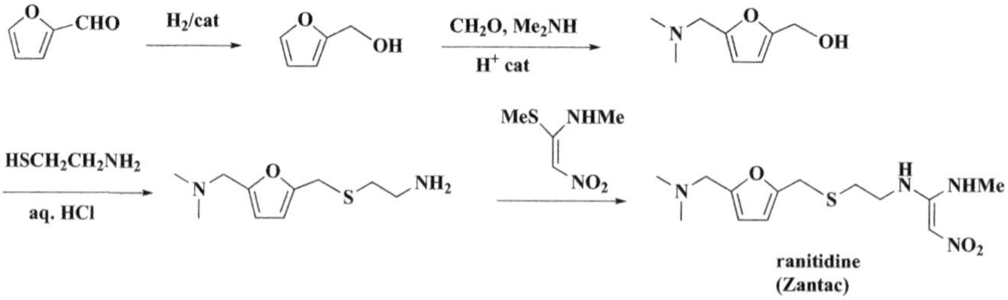

SCHEME 3.5 Synthesis of Zantac.

angiotensinogen into a decapeptide, angiotensin I. Angiotensin-converting enzyme (ACE) converts angiotensin I into angiotensin II (octapeptide), a potent vasoconstrictor, which causes an increase in blood pressure. Angiotensin II also helps release aldosterone, which is responsible for the retention of Na^+, K^+ ions, and water in the kidneys, leading to high blood pressure.

Two strategies were developed for the treatment of hypertension by inhibiting the RAS system. The first is the discovery of ACE inhibitors, such as captopril,[12] which are successfully used for the treatment of hypertension. The second strategy was the development of angiotensin II receptor antagonists, which inhibit the binding of angiotensin II to its AT1 and AT2 receptors. Losartan (Cozaar) is the first orally active angiotensin II receptor antagonist. Losartan is currently being investigated for the treatment of COVID-19.

The discovery of losartan[13a] began with the initial lead **1**, which was found to have weak antagonistic activity (Figure 3.15). Since no information on the structure of the receptor was available, based on computer modeling, it was concluded that a second carboxylic acid group in the molecule would improve potency. Compound **2** was synthesized, which showed ten-fold improvement in potency compared with initial lead **1**. Further modification of **2** led to compound **3**, which showed improvement in potency; however, it was not orally active. Introduction of a hydroxymethyl group on the imidazole ring and removal of the amide bond linker resulted in compound **4**, which was more lipophilic and orally active. Replacement of the carboxylic acid group on the aromatic ring with a tetrazole isostere led to the discovery of losartan. Losartan was 1000 times more potent than the initial lead **1** and was orally active, with a longer duration of action as an angiotensin II receptor antagonist. Later, it was found that both losartan ($t_{1/2} = 2h$) and its active metabolite **5** ($t_{1/2} = 6h$) were responsible for the long-lasting antihypertensive activity (Figures 3.15 and 3.16). Subsequent research showed that the binding of angiotensin II to its AT1 receptor caused vascular constriction, and binding to the AT2 receptor had no effect. Losartan selectively binds to the AT1 receptor. Losartan's structure has served as a prototype

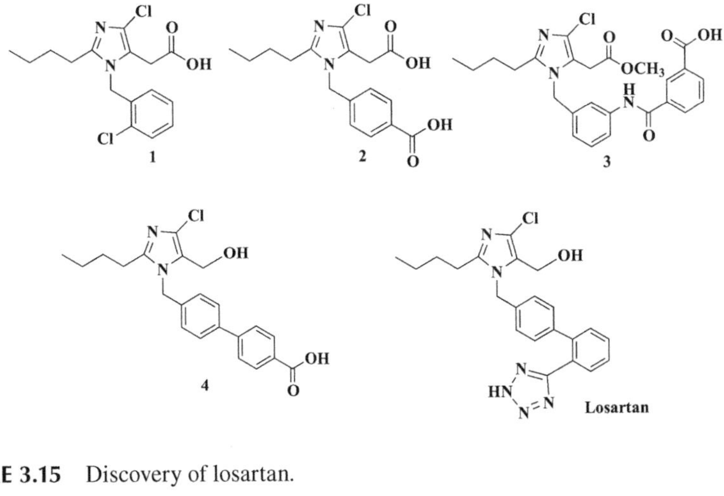

FIGURE 3.15   Discovery of losartan.

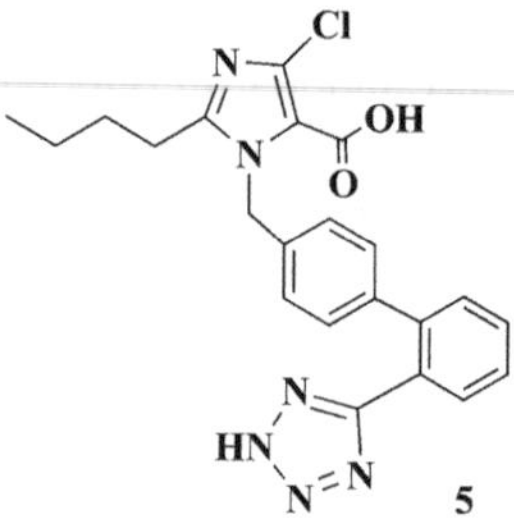

FIGURE 3.16 Metabolite of losartan.

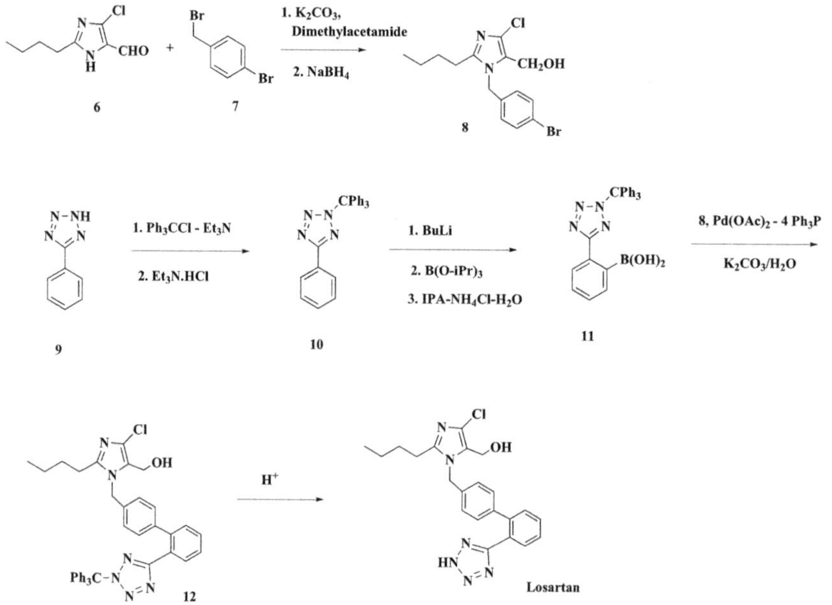

SCHEME 3.6 Synthesis of losartan.

for the discovery of several newer selective AT1 receptor antagonists for the treatment of hypertension.

The synthesis of losartan is shown in Scheme 3.6.[13b]

3.6 STEROIDS

Steroids were first isolated from mammalian sources and are produced in the adrenal glands, ovaries, and testes. Steroids are represented by tetracyclic rigid structures with several centers of asymmetry, are optically active, and represent single

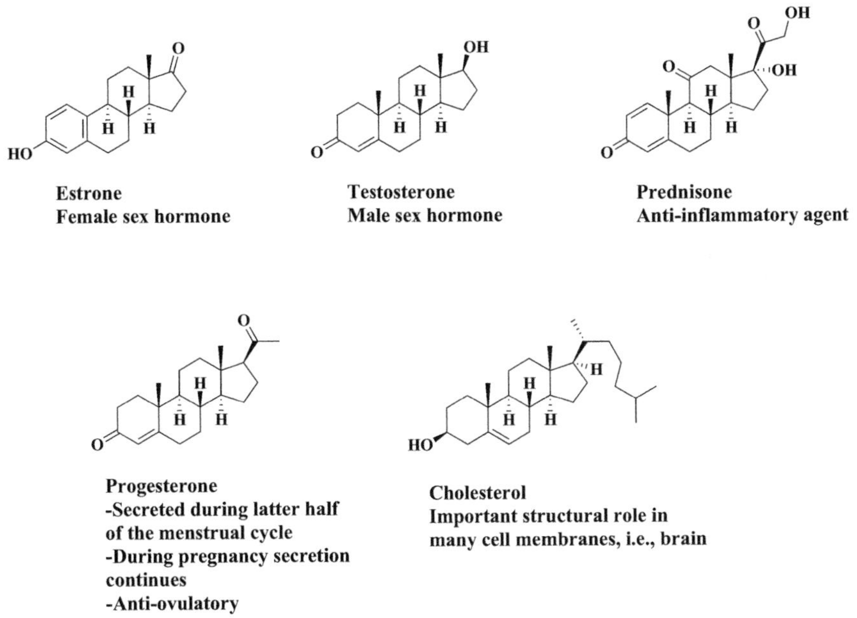

Estrone
Female sex hormone

Testosterone
Male sex hormone

Prednisone
Anti-inflammatory agent

Progesterone
**-Secreted during latter half
of the menstrual cycle
-During pregnancy secretion
continues
-Anti-ovulatory**

Cholesterol
**Important structural role in
many cell membranes, i.e., brain**

FIGURE 3.17 Examples of steroids and their biological role.

enantiomers (Figure 3.17). They are classified as sex hormones, such as estrone, testosterone, and progesterone, and corticosteroids, such as cortisone, prednisone, betamethasone, and dexamethasone. Much of the work on steroids was done from 1950 to 1960. Although this is presently not an active area of research, steroids continue to be used extensively as contraceptives and anti-inflammatory agents and in the treatment of cancer, autoimmune diseases, and, very recently, COVID-19.

3.6.1 Biosynthesis of Steroids

Mevalonic acid is the precursor for the biosynthesis of steroids[14] and terpenes. It is derived from acetyl coenzyme A as outlined in Scheme 3.7.

The conversion of mevalonic acid to squalene is shown in Scheme 3.8.

The conversion of squalene to lanosterol is shown in Scheme 3.9.

The conversion of lanosterol to cholesterol represents biosynthetic steps that are similar to those seen in the conversion to other steroids (Scheme 3.10).

3.6.2 Synthesis of Steroids

Diosgenin is obtained from the tubers of the wild yam (*Dioscorea villosa*), which is also known as kokoro. All clinically used steroids can be derived from it using appropriate chemical conversions. It should be noted that diosgenin possesses four rings with proper stereochemistry, as found in all steroids, and the rest of

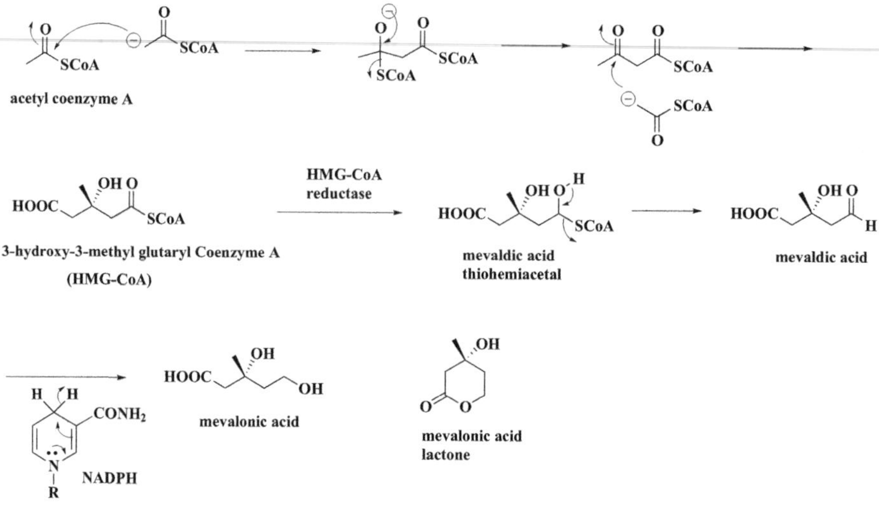

acetyl coenzyme A

3-hydroxy-3-methyl glutaryl Coenzyme A
(HMG-CoA)

HMG-CoA
reductase

mevaldic acid
thiohemiacetal

mevaldic acid

HOOC — OH (mevalonic acid)

mevalonic acid

mevalonic acid
lactone

NADPH

SCHEME 3.7   Biosynthesis of mevalonic acid from acetyl coenzyme A.

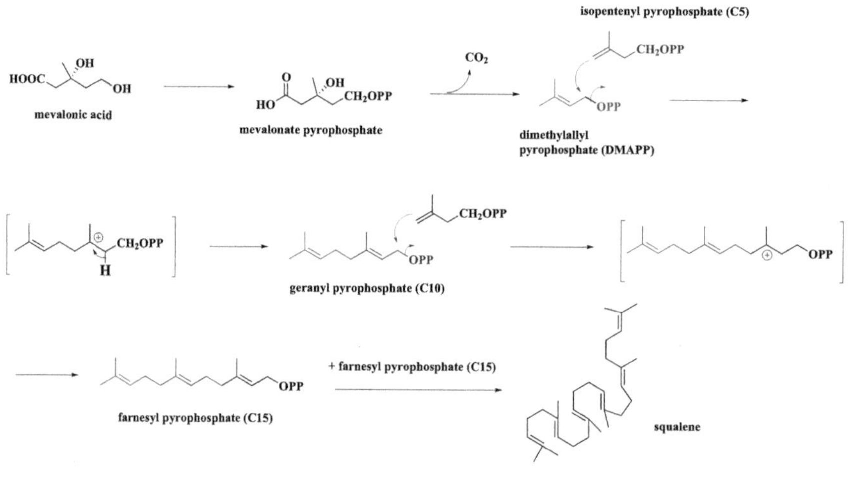

mevalonic acid

mevalonate pyrophosphate

isopentenyl pyrophosphate (C5)

dimethylallyl
pyrophosphate (DMAPP)

geranyl pyrophosphate (C10)

farnesyl pyrophosphate (C15)

+ farnesyl pyrophosphate (C15)

squalene

SCHEME 3.8   Biosynthesis of squalene from mevalonic acid.

the molecule is amenable to changes required for the synthesis of different steroids. Although total synthesis of steroids has been achieved, contributing much
knowledge to the chemical literature, however it has not reached commercial
significance. The synthesis of a few clinically important steroids is presented in
Schemes 3.11–3.14.

Testosterone[16] is synthesized from diosgenin as shown in Scheme 3.13. It is
metabolized in the liver and is not orally active. In the clinic, testosterone esters are

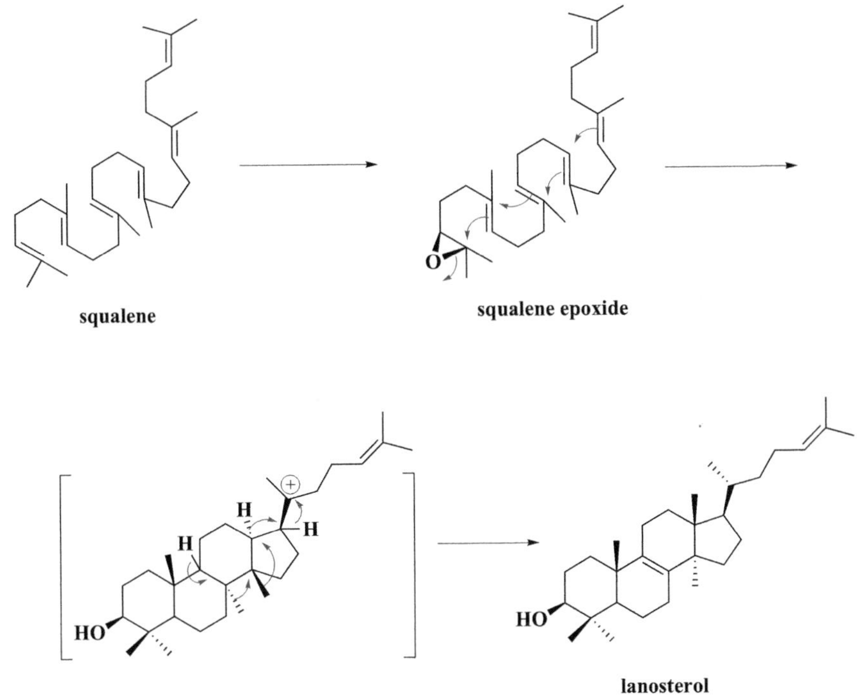

SCHEME 3.9   Biosynthesis of squalene to lanosterol.

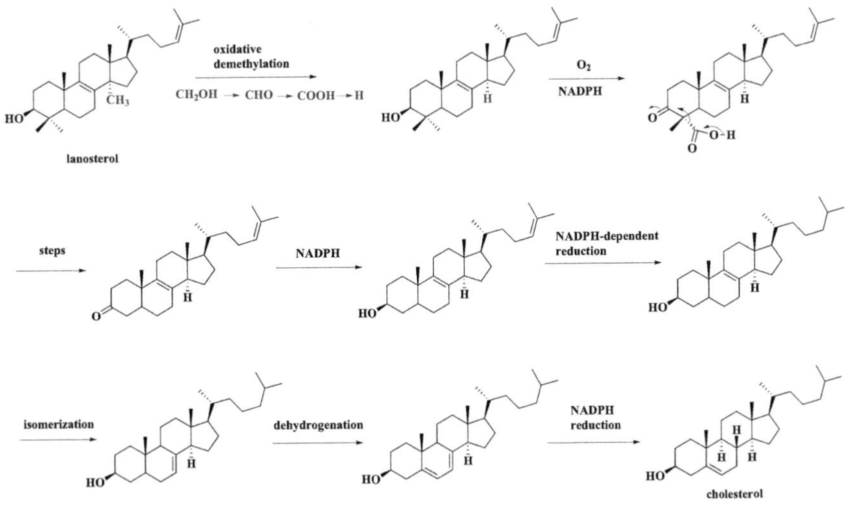

SCHEME 3.10   Biosynthesis of lanosterol to cholesterol.

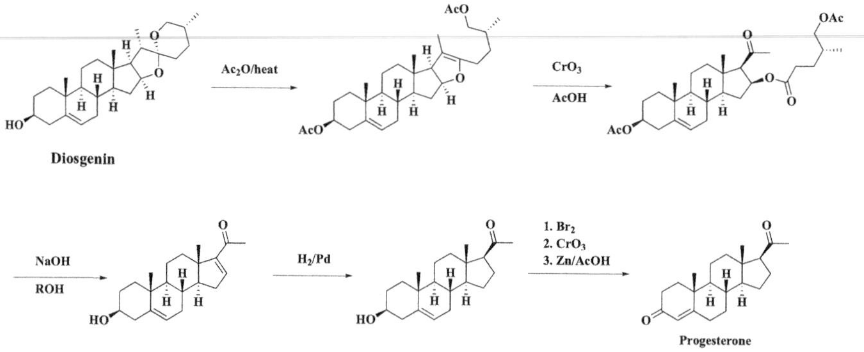

SCHEME 3.11   Synthesis of progesterone (Marker degradation).[15]

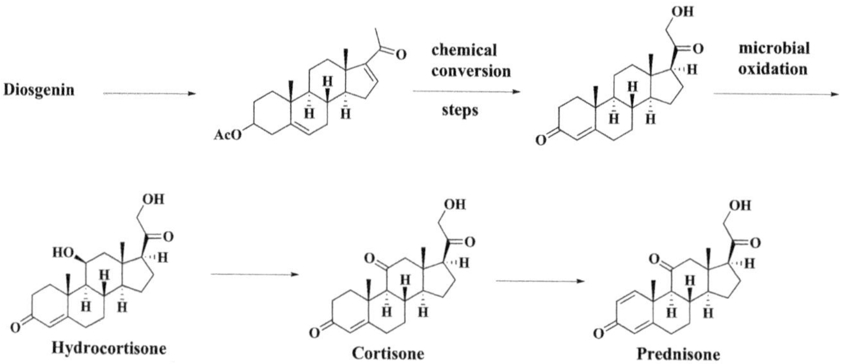

SCHEME 3.12   Synthesis of corticosteroids.

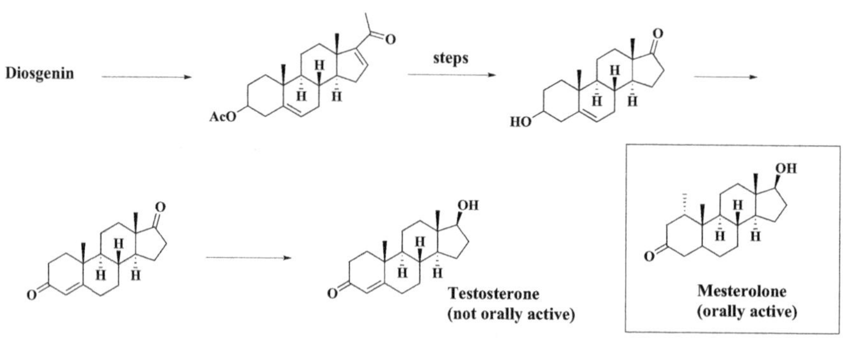

SCHEME 3.13   Synthesis of testosterone.

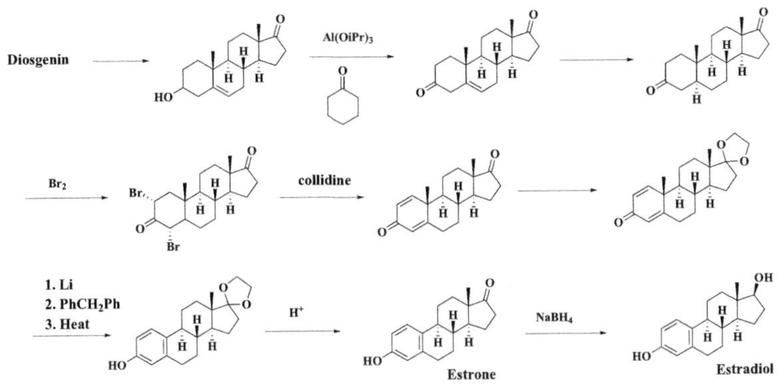

SCHEME 3.14 Synthesis of estrone and estradiol.

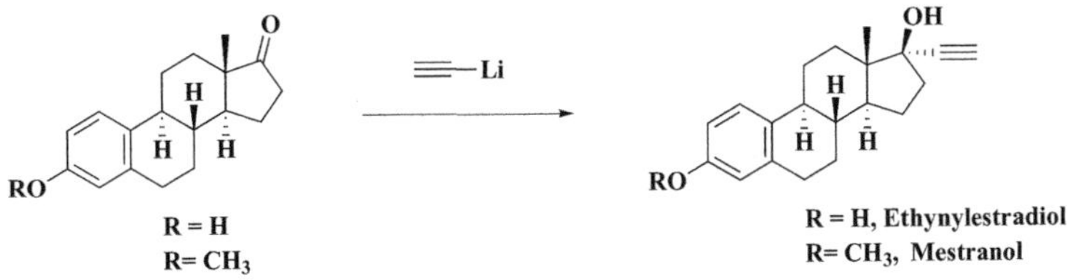

SCHEME 3.15 Synthesis of ethynylestradiol and mestranol.

used as injectables. An orally active synthetic testosterone derivative, mesterolone, is also used in the clinic.

Estrone is poorly absorbed orally and is metabolized by cytochrome P450 enzymes into several hydroxyestrones, which are eliminated as conjugates using sulfotransferases and glucuronidases. Substitution at the 17 position provides metabolically more stable derivatives, such as ethynylestradiol and mestranol (Scheme 3.15).

3.6.3 PROGESTERONE RECEPTOR ANTAGONISTS

Progesterone receptor (PR) is an intracellular steroidal receptor. PR antagonists[17] are used as contraceptives and for the treatment of tumors, uterine fibroids, and endometriosis. All clinically available PR antagonists (Figure 3.18) are steroids.

Perhaps one of the most well-known contraceptives is mifepristone (RU-486),[18] the structure and synthesis of which are shown in Scheme 3.16.

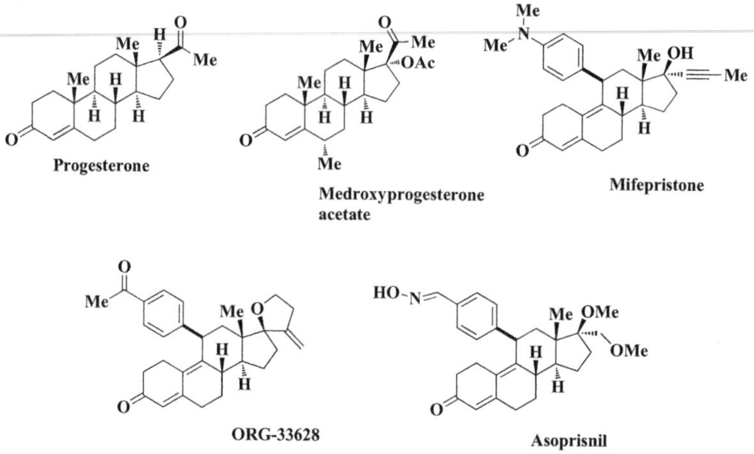

FIGURE 3.18 Clinically available progesterone receptor antagonists.

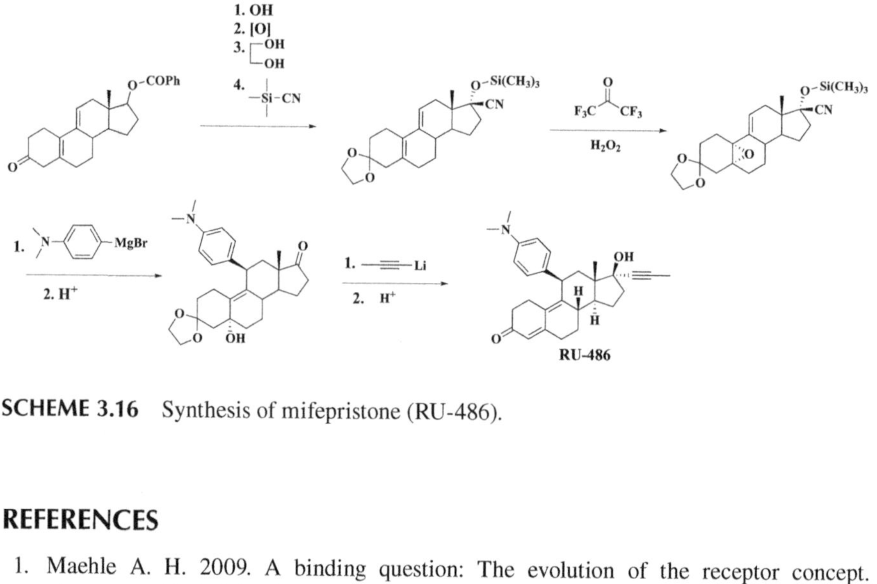

SCHEME 3.16 Synthesis of mifepristone (RU-486).

REFERENCES

1. Maehle A. H. 2009. A binding question: The evolution of the receptor concept. *Endeavour* 33(4):135–140.
2. (a) Sriram, K., and Insel, P. A. 2018. G protein-coupled receptors as targets for approved drugs: How many targets and how many drugs? *Mol. Pharmacol.* 93(4):251–258. (b) Rosenbaum, D., Rasmussen, S., and Kobilka, B. 2009. The structure and function of G-protein-coupled receptors. *Nature* 459:356–363. (c) Lappano, R., and Maggiolini, M. G. 2011. Protein-coupled receptors: Novel targets for drug discovery in cancer. *Nat. Rev. Drug Discov.* 10:47–60.
3. (a) Ing. H. R. 1963. Drug-receptor interaction. *Pure Appl. Chem.* 3(3):227–232. (b) Silverman, R. B. 2004. *Receptors: The Organic Chemistry of Drug Design and Drug Action*, 2nd ed., Elsevier Academic Press, Cambridge, Chap. 3, pp. 121–172.
4. (a) Nguyen, L. A., He, H., and Pham-Huy, C. 2006. Chiral drugs: An overview. *Int. J. Biomed. Sci.* 2(2):85–100. (b) Brooks, W. H., Guida, W. C., and Daniel, K. G. 2011.

The significance of chirality in drug design and development. *Curr. Top Med. Chem.* 11(7):760–770.

5. (a) Best, C. H., Dale, H. H., Dudley, H. W., and Thorpe, W. V. 1927. The nature of the Vaso-dilator constituents of certain tissue extracts. *J. Physiol.* 62(4):397–417. (b) Parsons, M. E., and Ganellin, C. R. 2006. Histamine and its receptors. *Br. J. Pharmacol.* 147(Suppl 1):S127–S135.

6. (a) Thurmond, R., Gelfand, E., and Dunford, P. 2008. The role of histamine H1 and H4 receptors in allergic inflammation: The search for new antihistamines. *Nat. Rev. Drug Discov.* 7:41–53. (b) Leurs, R., Smit, M. J., and Timmerman, H. 1995. Molecular pharmacological aspects of histamine receptors. *Pharmac. Ther.* 66:413–463.

7. (a) Villani, F. J., Magatti, C. V., Vashi, D. B., et al. 1986. N-substituted 11-(4-piperidy lene)-5,6-dihydro-11H-benzo-[5,6]cyclohepta [1,2-b]pyridines. Antihistamines with no sedating liability. *Arzneimittelforschung.* 36(9):1311–1314. (b) Motasim Billah, M., Egan, R. W., Ganguly, A. K., et al. 1991. Discovery and preliminary pharmacology of Sch 37370, a dual antagonist of PAF and histamine. *Lipids* 26:1172–1174.

8. (a) Piwinski, J. J., Wong, J. K., Green M. J., et al. 1991. Dual antagonists of platelet-activating factor and histamine. Identification of structural requirements for dual activity of N-acyl-4-(5,6-dihydro-11H-benzo[5,6]cyclohepta[1,2-b]pyridin-11-ylidene) piperidines. *J. Med. Chem.* 34(1):457–461. (b) Piwinski, J. J., Wong, J. K., Chan, T. M., et al. 1990. Hydroxylated metabolites of loratadine: An example of conformational dia-stereomers due to atropisomerism. *J. Org. Chem.* 55(10):3341–3350.

9. Kawai, S. H., Hambalek, R. J., and Just, G. 1994. A facile synthesis of an oxidation prod-uct of Terfenadine. *J. Org. Chem.* 59(9):2620–2622.

10. (a) Brimblecombe, R. W., Duncan, W. A. M., Durant, G. J., et al. 1978. Characterization and development of cimetidine as a histamine H2 receptor antagonist. *Gasteroenterology* 74:339–347. (b) Molinder, H. K. 1994. The development of cimetidine: 1964–1976. A human story. *J. Clin. Gastroenterol.* 19(3):248–254.

11. Glushkov, R. G., Adamskaya, E. V., Vosyakova, T. I., et al. 1990. Pathways of synthesis of ranitidine (review). *Pharm. Chem. J.* 24:369–373.

12. (a) Cushman, D., and Ondetti, M. A. 1999. Design of angiotensin converting enzyme inhibitors. *Nat. Med.* 5:1110–1112. (b) Cushman, D. W. and Ondetti, M. A. 1991. History of the design of captopril and related inhibitors of angiotensin converting enzyme. *Hypertension* 17(4):589–592.

13. (a) Larsen, R. D., King, A. O., Chen, C. Y. 1994. Efficient synthesis of Losartan, a non-peptide angiotensin II receptor antagonist. *J. Org. Chem.* 59:6391–6394. (b) Carini, D. J., Duncia, J. V., Aldrich, P. E., et al. 1991. Nonpeptide angiotensin II receptor antagonists: The discovery of a series of N-(Biphenylylmethyl)imidazoles as potent, orally active antihypertensives. *J. Med. Chem.* 34:2525–2547.

14. (a) Cornforth, J. W., and Popjak, G. 1958. Biosynthesis of cholesterol. *Br. Med. Bull.* 14(3):221–225. (b) Popjak, G., and Cornforth, J. W. 1960. The biosynthesis of cholesterol. *Adv. Enzymol. Relat. Subj. Biochem.* 22:281–335.

15. (a) Marker, R. E., and Rohrmann, E. 1939. Sterols. LXXXI. Conversion of sarsasapo-genin to pregnanediol-3(α),20(α). *J. Am. Chem. Soc.* 61(12):3592–3593. (b) Lehmann, P. A., Bolivar, A. G., and Quintero R. R. 1973. Russel E. Marker. Pioneer of the Mexican steroid industry. *J. Chem. Educ.* 50(3):195–199.

16. Marker, R. E. 1940. Stereols. CV. The preparation of testosterone and related compounds from sarsasapogenin and diosgenin. *J. Am. Chem. Soc.* 62(9):2543–2547.

17. Spitz, I. M. 2006. Progesterone receptor antagonists. *Curr. Opin. Investig. Drugs* 7(10):882–890.

18. Hazra, B. G., and Pore, V. S. 2001. Mifepristone (RU-486), the recently developed anti-progesterone drug and its analogues. *J. Indian Inst. Sci.* 81:287–298.

4 Anticancer Drugs

The discovery of anticancer drugs follows largely the pathways described for the discovery of other classes of drugs. For example, the process includes enzyme inhibitors such as farnesyl protein transferase for the treatment of lung cancer and receptor antagonists such as tamoxifen. Natural products such as Taxol are in use for the treatment of cancer.

4.1 EXAMPLES OF ANTICANCER DRUGS FROM PLANTS

Vinca alkaloids[1a] (Figure 4.1) from *Catharanthus roseus*, or *Vinca rosea* (Madagascar periwinkle), were originally thought to be useful as antidiabetic drugs; however, in animal experiments they showed no effect in reducing blood sugar. The purified active components (i.e., vinblastine and vincristine) showed activity as anticancer agents. Treatment of vinblastine with ammonia in methanol yielded the anticancer drug vindesine (Scheme 4.1),[1b] which is used for the treatment of non-small cell lung cancer, leukemia, testicular cancer, and non-Hodgkin's lymphoma.

4.1.1 MECHANISM OF ANTICANCER ACTIVITY OF VINCRISTINE

During cell division (mitosis) the two developing daughter cells are held together by thin fibers called microtubules. These are polymers based on a protein known as tubulin. Tubulin is a dimer of the α and β subunits. These associate to from heteroduplexes, which then join together as a "head to tail" function. The resulting

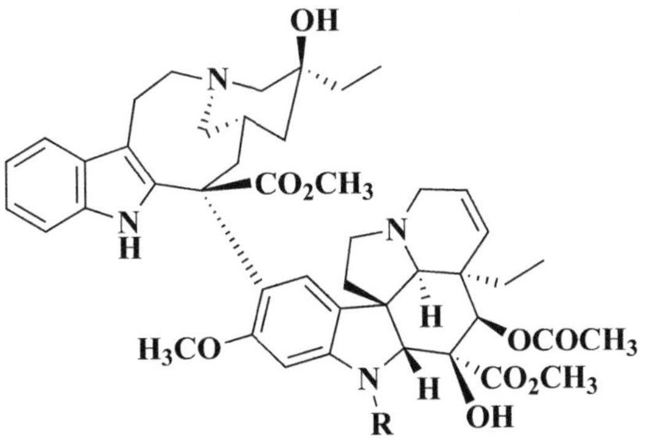

Vinblastine R = CH$_3$
Vincristine R = CHO

FIGURE 4.1 Structure of *Vinca* alkaloids.

DOI: 10.1201/9781003182573-4

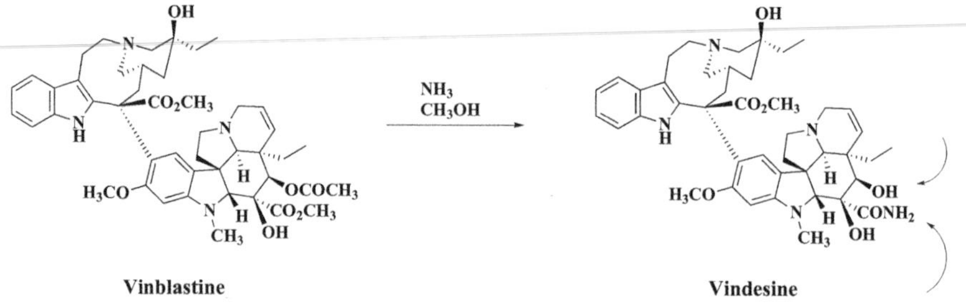

SCHEME 4.1 Chemical conversion of vinblastine to vindesine.

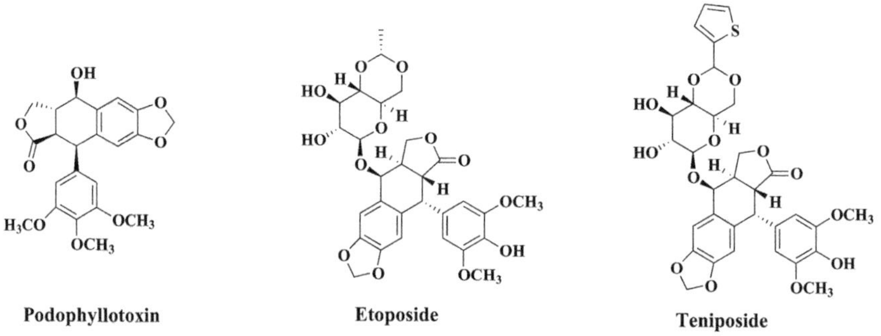

FIGURE 4.2 Structure of anticancer compounds.

filaments then polymerize to form microtubules. In the presence of *Vinca* alkaloids, the existing microtubules break down to produce tubulin subunit pairs. The subunit pairs bind to the drug, and the complex prevents the formation of microtubules. Cell division does not occur, immature cells die, and cell proliferation ceases.

Podophyllotoxin[2] is obtained from the Himalayan plant *Podophyllum emodi* (Figure 4.2). Newer analogs i.e., etoposide[3] and teniposide[4]) are used in the treatment of testicular cancer, Hodgkin's disease, etc.

Taxol[5a] is extracted from the English yew (*Taxus baccata*) and Pacific yew (*Taxus brevifolia*), and its structure was elucidated using x-ray crystallography (Figure 4.3). Taxol prevents cell division by stabilizing microtubule assembly, which leads to cell death.[5c,5d] The development of Taxol as an anticancer agent was challenging because of the difficulty of isolating it in sufficient quantities from the bark of yew trees. For example, only 500 mg of Taxol is obtained from 12 kg of yew tree bark. Additionally, it is rather insoluble, making delivery of the drug very difficult.

A clinical trial of Taxol began in 1983, and in 1989 its efficacy in ovarian cancer was confirmed. It was approved in 1992 for the treatment of ovarian cancer and was approved later on for the treatment of metastatic breast cancer and lung cancer. However, its use was restricted due to the lack of availability of the drug prior to the discovery of Taxotere.[6] The precursor to Taxotere is 10-deacetylbaccatin III, which is extracted from the needles of yew trees. A total of 1 g of the Taxotere precursor

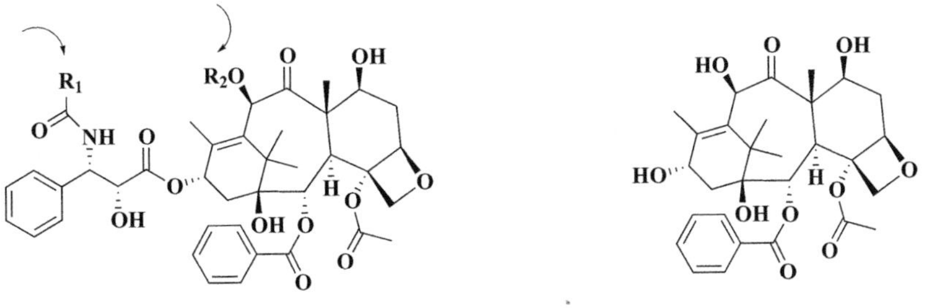

Taxol R₁= Ph, R₂= COCH₃
Taxotere R₁= Ot-Bu, R₂= H

10-deacetylbaccatin III

FIGURE 4.3   Structure of Taxol, Taxotere, and 10-deactylbaccatin III.

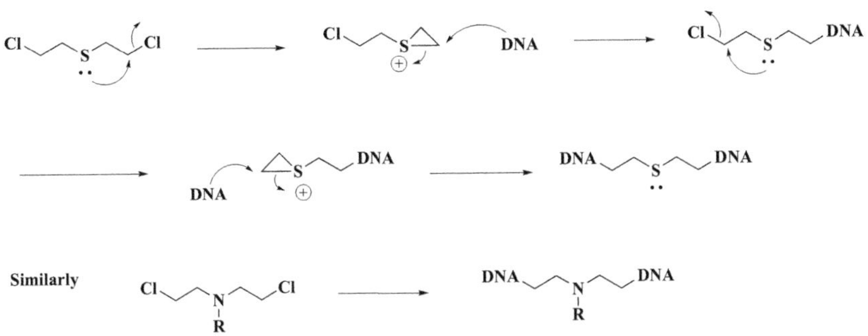

SCHEME 4.2   Mechanism of alkylation by mustard reagents.

can be obtained from 3 kg of needles without sacrificing the trees. In addition, the solubility characteristics of Taxotere are far superior to those of Taxol. With these developments, Taxotere became a very important addition to anticancer therapy.

4.2 DNA ALKYLATING AGENTS

Several alkylating agents[7] were discovered during the Second World War and are still in use as chemotherapeutic agents. In the process of killing cancer cells, they also kill normal cells, thus resulting in toxicity. The general mechanism of activity of these DNA alkylating agents can be explained using the example of mustard reagents (Scheme 4.2).

Cisplatin[8] is an alkylating agent and is used for the treatment of testicular, lung, and bladder cancer. Its mechanism of action is similar to that of mustard reagents. Examples of a few other alkylating agents are shown in Figure 4.4.

Duocarmycins are another class of DNA alkylating agents[9] that are isolated from the culture broth of *Streptomyces* bacteria (Figure 4.5). These compounds are very potent as antitumor agents. Duocarmycins possess a cyclopropane ring in their core structure, which helps to alkylate adenine at the N3 position.

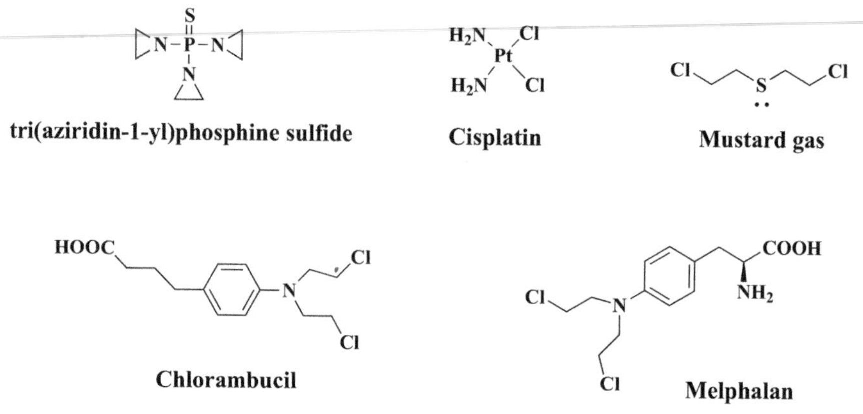
tri(aziridin-1-yl)phosphine sulfide
Cisplatin
Mustard gas
Chlorambucil
Melphalan

FIGURE 4.4 Examples of alkylating agents.

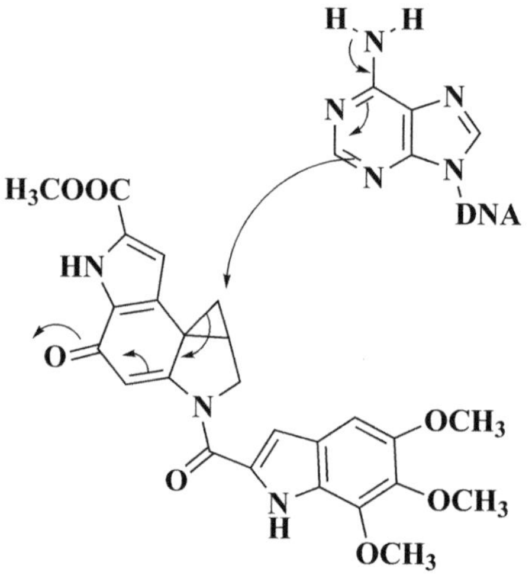
DNA
H3COOC
OCH3
OCH3
OCH3

FIGURE 4.5 Mechanism of DNA alkylation on duocarmycin.

4.3 ANTIMETABOLITES

The structure of the cytotoxic agent methotrexate[10] bears similarities to that of folic acid (Figure 4.6), and it found use in the treatment of breast and lung cancer as well as other forms of cancer. It is also used for the treatment of autoimmune diseases such as psoriasis and rheumatoid arthritis. Methotrexate is synthesized as shown in Scheme 4.3.

To avoid the metabolic degradation of methotrexate, edatrexate was synthesized (Scheme 4.4).

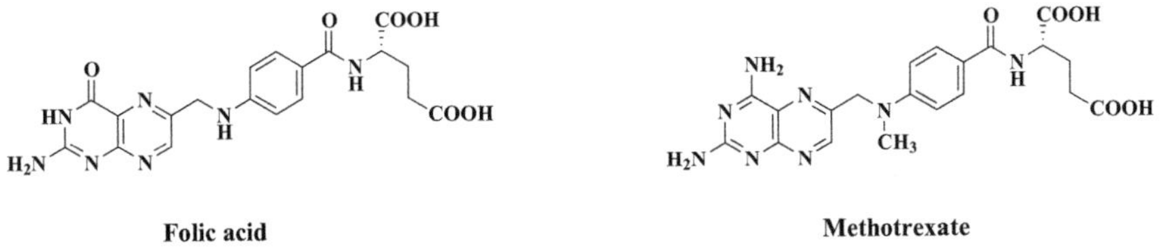

FIGURE 4.6 Structure of folic acid and methotrexate.

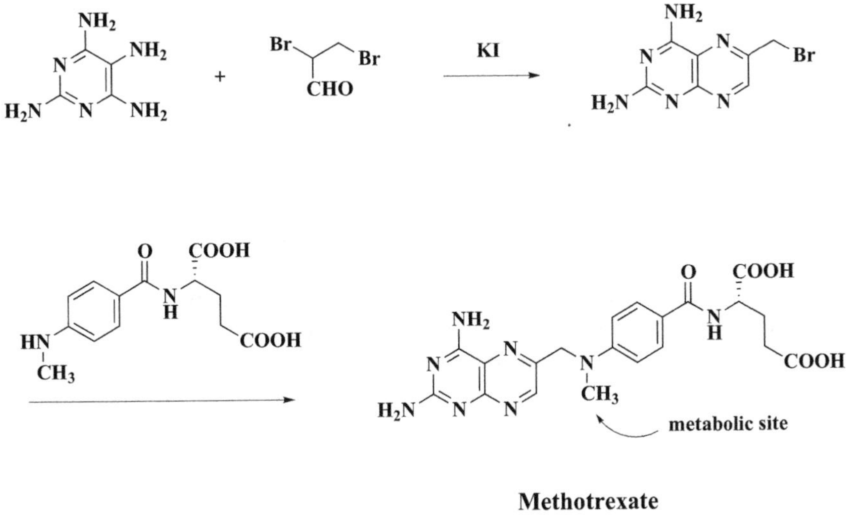

SCHEME 4.3 Synthesis of methotrexate.

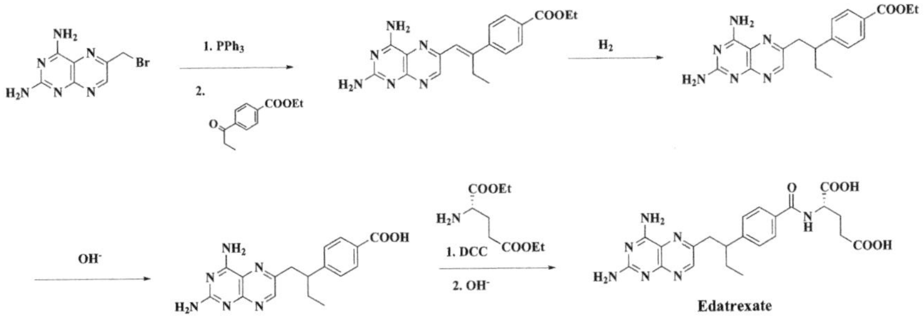

SCHEME 4.4 Synthesis of edatrexate.

4.4 ESTROGEN RECEPTOR ANTAGONISTS

Tamoxifen[11] is commonly used for the treatment of breast cancer. Most breast cancers need supplies of estrone to grow. Estrone attaches to the estrogen receptor on cancer cells and sends signals for cellular proliferation; when it is unregulated, it causes cancer. ER-positive patients respond very well to tamoxifen, which attaches to the estrogen receptor but does not cause the cells to divide. It also does not allow estrone to occupy the receptor. Clomiphene is a close analog of tamoxifen and is also primarily used for the treatment of breast cancer (Scheme 4.5).

4.5 AROMATASE INHIBITORS

Aromatase is a P450 oxidative enzyme that converts androstenedione to estrone (Scheme 4.6). Examples of potent aromatase inhibitors[12] are shown in Figure 4.7.

4.6 KINASE INHIBITORS

Protein kinases[13] are the largest superfamily of enzymes and play an important role in cellular functions, such as metabolism, signal transduction, survival, and differentiation. Malfunction or overexpression of protein kinases is found in many diseases, mostly tumors. Kinases are the enzymes involved in phosphorylation, which is an important mechanism for cell regulation. When a protein is phosphorylated, a gamma phosphate group from adenosine triphosphate (ATP) is transferred to the amino acid residue–containing -OH group (tyrosine, threonine, serine) on the target protein (Scheme 4.7).

Several classes of kinases are known based on the amino acid residue being phosphorylated, including protein tyrosine kinases, protein tyrosine kinase–like enzymes, and protein threonine/serine kinases. Currently, there are 52 FDA-approved drugs that target 20 different protein kinases, which represents a small fraction of the

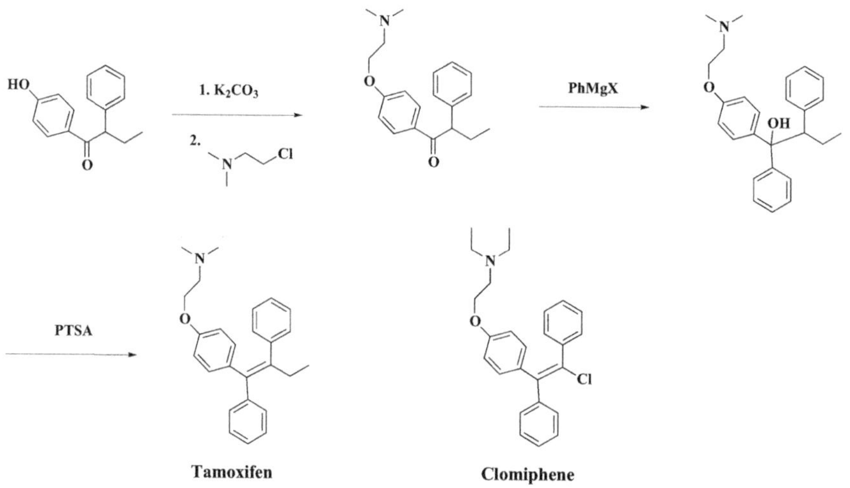

SCHEME 4.5 Synthesis of tamoxifen and its analog, clomiphene.

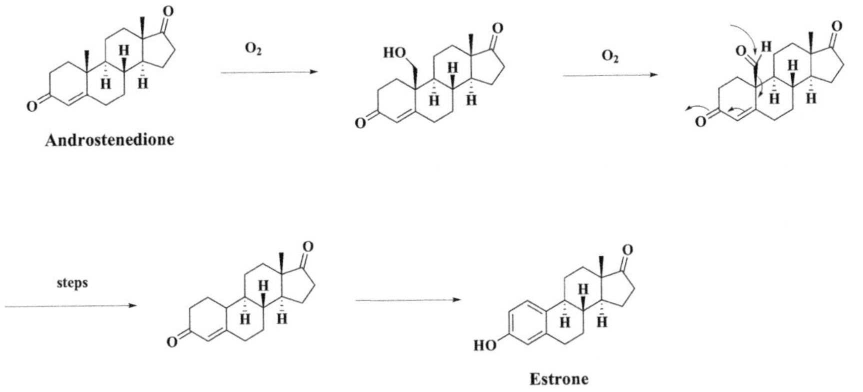

SCHEME 4.6 Conversion of androstenedione to estrone.

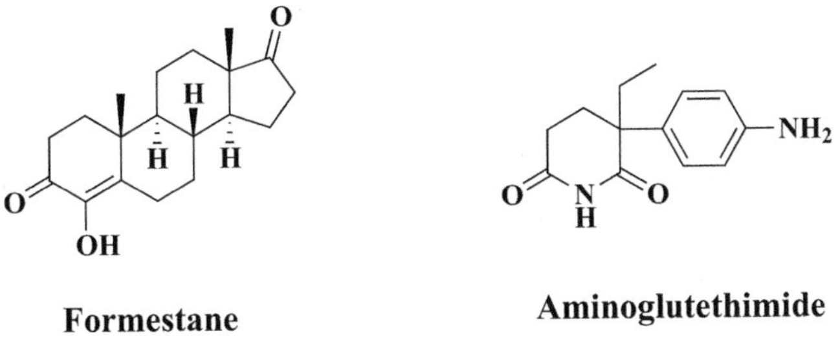

Formestane

Aminoglutethimide

FIGURE 4.7 Examples of aromatase inhibitors.

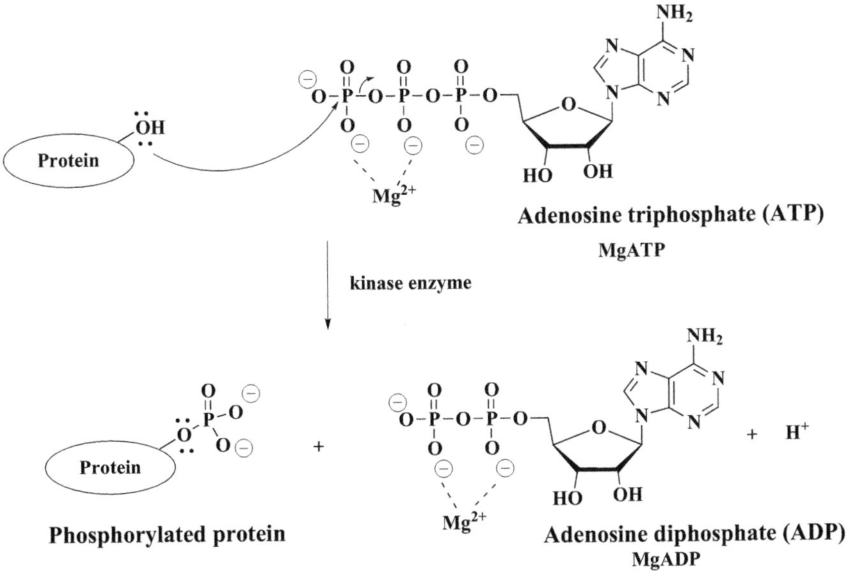

SCHEME 4.7 Mechanism of phosphorylation.

518-member protein kinase family. A few examples of drugs that target kinases are discussed in the following sections.

4.6.1 IMATINIB (GLEEVEC)

Chronic myeloid leukemia (CML) is a rare form of cancer in which bone marrow cells that give rise to white blood cells begin to divide faster than normal. CML is associated with chromosomal abnormalities wherein chromosome 22 is much shorter than normal and missing material is transferred to chromosome 9. The truncated 22 is known as the Philadelphia chromosome. The translocation event between 9 and 22 results in fusion of the two broken genes. The BCR gene on 9 and the ABL gene on 22 generate a new gene: BCR-ABL. The product of the BCR-ABL gene is a protein kinase. In normal cells this controls cell division and growth. The abnormal fusion protein retains the tyrosine kinase activity of ABL, but the signals are not regulated; thus, massive numbers of cells are produced. Gleevec[14] is specific to BCR-ABL tyrosine kinase and blocks the signal the abnormal protein generates (Scheme 4.8).

4.6.2 GEFITINIB (IRESSA)

Overexpression of the epidermal growth factor receptor (EGFR) is common in a wide variety of solid tumors, including non-small cell lung carcinoma and ovarian, bladder, and prostate carcinoma. Iressa[15] is an EGFR antagonist (Scheme 4.9). It blocks growth signals in cancer cells, which are mediated in part by the tyrosine kinases associated with EGFR.

4.6.3 BARICITINIB (OLUMIANT)

Baricitinib[16a] is an orally active selective Janus kinase (i.e., JAK1 and JAK2) inhibitor that is used for the treatment of rheumatoid arthritis. Janus kinases (i.e., JAK1,

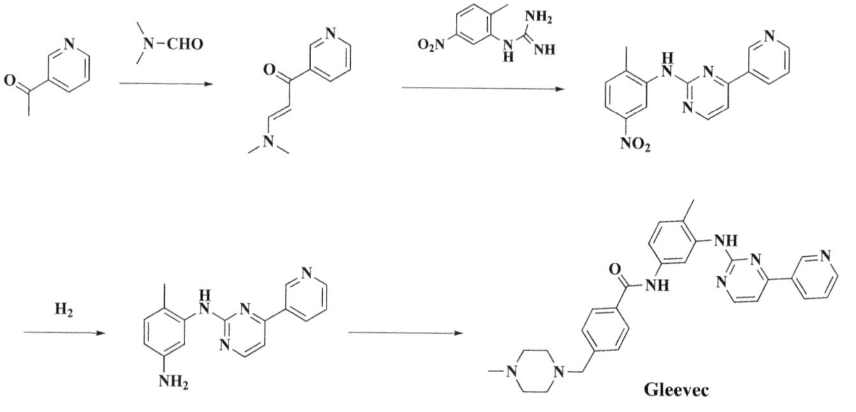

SCHEME 4.8   Synthesis of Gleevec.

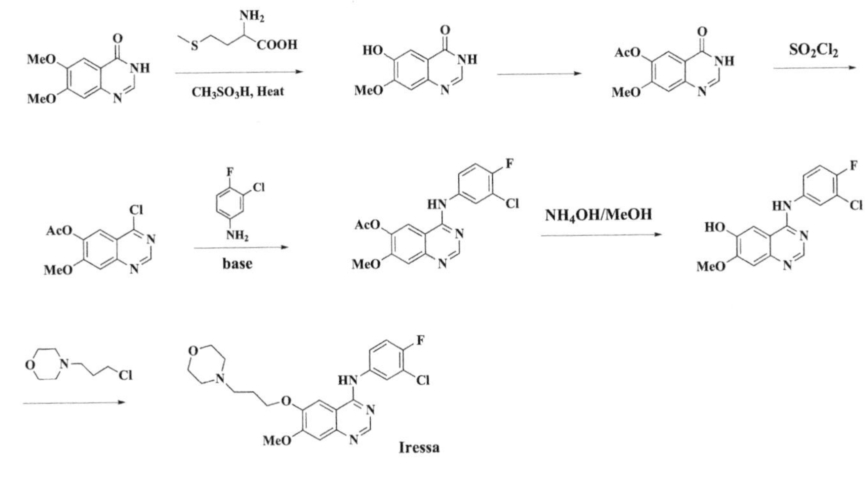

SCHEME 4.9   Synthesis of Iressa.

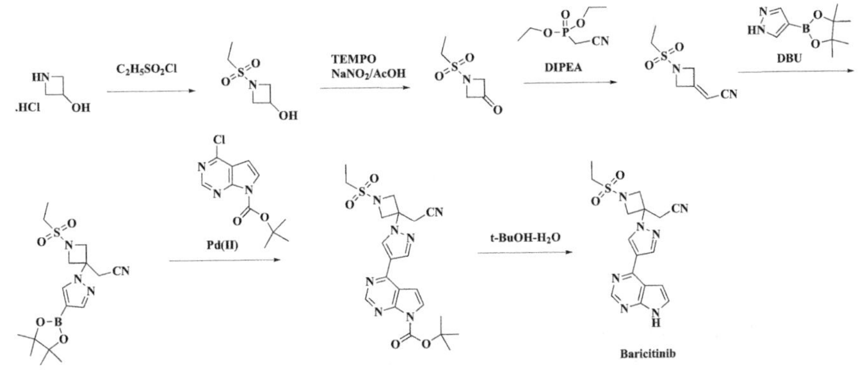

SCHEME 4.10   Synthesis of baricitinib.

JAK2, JAK3, TYK2) play a critical role in the regulation of immune and inflammatory responses. JAKs associate with the intracellular domain of cytokine receptors
type I and II and are activated upon ligand-induced receptor homo- or heterodimer-
ization, resulting in the phosphorylation of tyrosine residues within the cytoplasmic
domain of the receptors. These phosphorylated receptors serve as docking sites for
signal transducer and activator of transcription (STAT) proteins. The STATs are then
phosphorylated by the JAKs and translocate to the nucleus, where they act as transcription factors, regulating gene expression. Selective JAK inhibitors such as baricitinib control unwanted or overactive immune pathways. Baricitinib (Scheme 4.10)
in combination with the antiviral drug remdesivir was recently approved by the FDA
for the treatment of COVID-19.[16b]

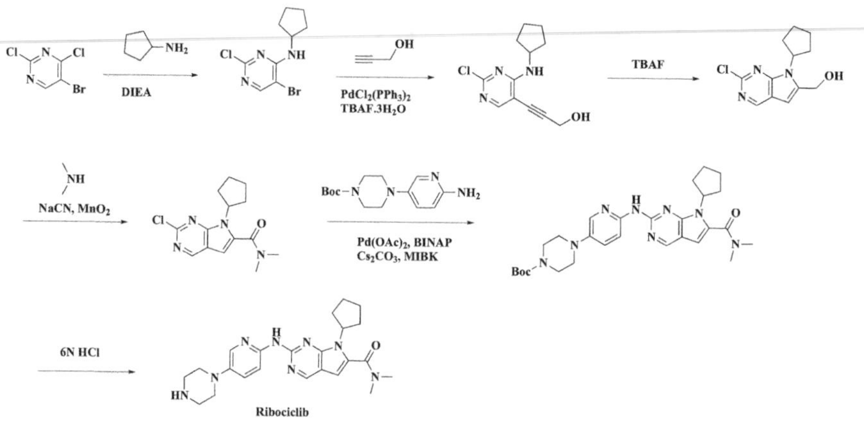

SCHEME 4.11   Synthesis of ribociclib.

4.6.4 RIBOCICLIB (KISQALI)

Cyclin-dependent kinases (CDKs) are serine/threonine protein kinases that play a primary role in the control of cell cycle progression. CDK inhibitors are hormone receptor–positive (HR+) and human epidermal growth factor receptor 2–negative (HER2-) in advanced breast cancer, and they work by selectively inhibiting CDK4/6 proteins and blocking the transition from the G1 to S phase of the cell cycle. The CDKs phosphorylate retinoblastoma (Rb) proteins, which are key proteins involved in regulating cell proliferation. Activation of the CDK-Rb pathway is common in breast cancer. By blocking this path, CDK4/6 inhibitors such as ribociclib[17] are able to block cell cycle progression in the middle of the G1 phase and prevent cancer cell progression. The synthesis of ribociclib is shown in Scheme 4.11.

4.6.5 ENTRECTINIB (ROZLYTREK)

Entrectinib[18] is a potent, orally available inhibitor of anaplastic lymphoma kinase (ALK), which is a receptor tyrosine kinase responsible for the development of various tumors. It has been prescribed for the treatment of solid tumors that have a neurotrophic tyrosine receptor kinase (NTRK) gene fusion without a known resistance mutation as well as ROS1-positive non-small cell lung cancer (NSLC). Using structure-based design, an initial lead compound (I), identified by high-throughput screening (HTS), was further optimized to yield entrectinib (Figure 4.8). It was found that an appropriate substitution at the 2' end of phenyl ring A, such as -NH-R, resulted in binding to the adenosine triphosphate (ATP) sugar pocket of the ALK active site while displacing the water molecule. This further resulted in stabilization of the conformation of the drug via the formation of an intramolecular hydrogen bond involving the hydrogen of the ortho amino group and the carbonyl of the adjacent carboxamide moiety. The synthesis of entrectinib is shown in Scheme 4.12.

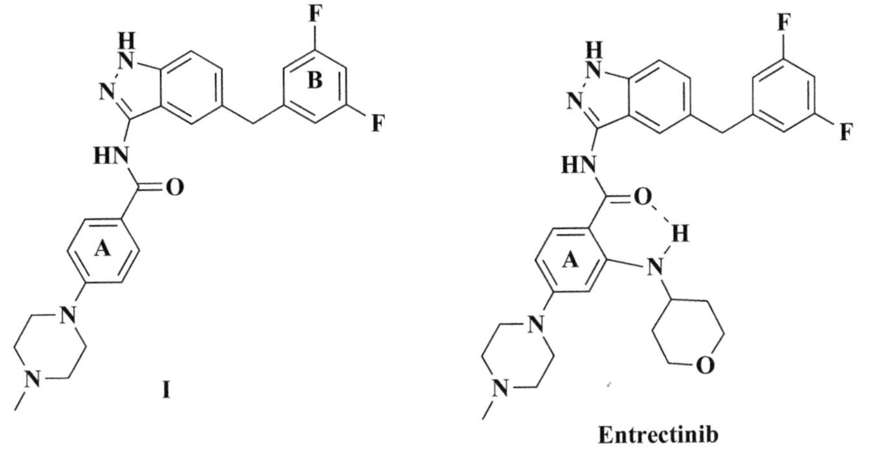

FIGURE 4.8 Structure of the initial lead (I) and entrectinib.

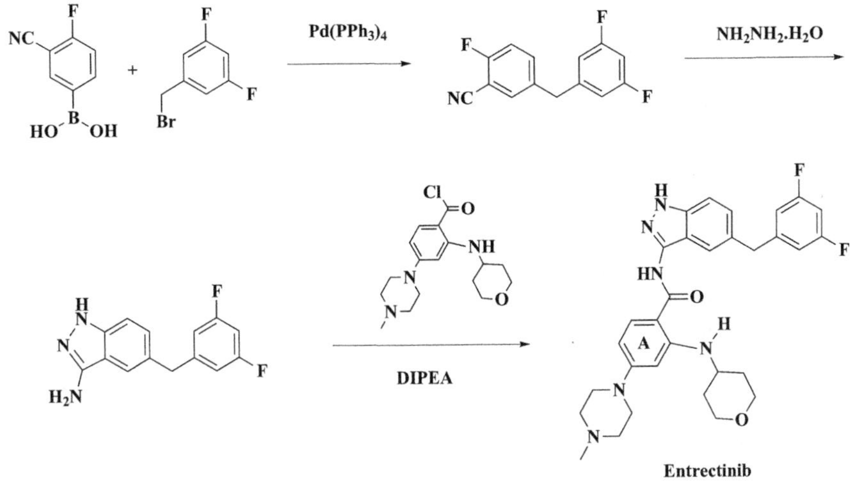

SCHEME 4.12 Synthesis of entrectinib.

REFERENCES

1. (a) Johnson, I. S., Armstrong, J. G., Gorman, M., et al. 1963. The Vinca alkaloids: A new class of oncolytic agents. *Cancer Res.* 23:1390–1427. (b) Keglevich, P., Hazai, L., Kalaus, G., et al. 2012. Modifications on the basic skeletons of vinblastine and vincristine. *Molecules* 17:5893–5914. (c) Himes, R. H., Kersey, R. N., Heller-Bettinger, I., et al. 1976. Action of the vinca alkaloids vincristine, vinblastine, and desacety vinblastine amide on microtubules in vitro. *Cancer Res.* 36:3798–3802. (d) Himes, R. H. 1991. Interactions of the catharanthus (Vinca) alkaloids with tubulin and microtubules. *Pharmacol Ther.* 51:257–267.

2. (a) Jackson, D. E., and Dewick, P. M. 1985. Tumor-inhibitory aryltetralin lignans from Podophyllum pleianthum. *Phytochemistry* 24:2407–2409. (b) You, Y. 2005. Podophyllotoxin derivatives: Current synthetic approaches for new anticancer agents. *Curr. Pharm. Des.* 11(13):1695–1717.

3. (a) Bromberg, K. D., Burgin, A. B., and Osheroff, N. 2003. A two-drug model for etoposide action against human topoisomerase IIα. *J. Biol. Chem.* 278(9):7406–7412. (b) Hande, K. R. 1998. Etoposide: Four decades of development of a topoisomerase II inhibitor. *Eur J Cancer* 34:1514–1521.

4. Long, B. H. 1992. Mechanism of action of teniposide (VM-26) and comparison with etoposide (VP-16). *Semin. Oncol.* 19:3–19.

5. (a) Nicolaou, K. C., and Sorensen, E. J. 2014. *Classics in Total Synthesis*, 6th ed., Wiley-VCH, Weinheim. (b) Wani, M. C., Taylor, H. L., Wall, M. E., et al. 1971. Plant antitumor agents. VI. Isolation and structure of Taxol, a novel antileukemic and antitumor agent from Taxus breyifolia. *J. Am. Chem. Soc.* 93(9):2325–2327. (c) Schiff, P. C., and Horwitz, S. B. 1980. Taxol stabilizes microtubules in mouse fibroblast cells. *Proc. Natl. Acad. Sci.* (USA) 77:1561–1565. (d) Parness, J., and Horwitz, S. B. 1981. Taxol binds to polymerized tubulin in vitro. *J. Cell Biol.* 91:479–487. (e) Kanda, Y., Nakamura, H., Umemiya, S., et al. 2020. Two-phase synthesis of Taxol. *J. Am. Chem. Soc.* 142(23):10526–10533.

6. Guenard, D., Gueritte-Voegelein, F., and Potier, P. 1993. Taxol and Taxotere: Discovery, chemistry, and structure-activity relationships. *Acc. Chem. Res.* 26(4):160–167.

7. Warwick. G. P. 1963. The mechanism of action of alkylating agents. *Cancer Res.* 23:1315–1333.

8. Wiltshaw, E. 1979. Cisplatin in the treatment of cancer: The first metal antitumor drug. *Platinum Metals Rev.* 23(3):90–98.

9. Boger, D. L., and Johnson, D. S. 1995. CC-1065 and the duocarmycins: Unraveling the keys to a new class of naturally derived DNA alkylating agents. *Proc. Natl. Acad. Sci.* 92:3642–3649. (b) Yamada, K., Kurokawa, T., Tokuyama, H., et. al. 2003. Total synthesis of the Duocarmycins. *J. Am. Chem. Soc.* 125(22):6630–6631.

10. (a) Cronstein, B. N., and Aune, T. M. 2020. Methotrexate and its mechanisms of action in inflammatory arthritis. *Nat Rev Rheumatol* 16:145–154. (b) Raimondi, M. V., Randazzo, O., La Franca, M., et al. 2019. DHFR inhibitors: Reading the past for discovering novel anticancer agents. *Molecules.* 24(6):1140.

11. (a) Jordan, V. C. 2006. Tamoxifen (ICI46,474) as a targeted therapy to treat and prevent breast cancer. *Br. J. Pharmacol.* 147:S269–S276. (b) Jordan, V. C. 1998. Antiestrogenic action of raloxifene and tamoxifen: Today and tomorrow. *J. Natl. Cancer Inst.* 90(13):967–971. (c) Quirke, V. M. 2017. Tamoxifen from failed contraceptive pill to best-selling breast cancer medicine: A case-study in pharmaceutical innovation. *Front. Pharmacol.* 8:620.

12. (a) Wiseman, L. R., and McTavish, D. 1993. Formestane. *Drugs* 45:66–84. (b) Fabian, C. J. 2007. The what, why and how of aromatase inhibitors: Hormonal agents for treatment and prevention of breast cancer. *Int. J. Clin. Prac.* 61(12):2051–2063.

13. Roskoski Jr., R. 2020. Properties of FDA approved small molecule protein kinase inhibitors: A 2020 update. *Pharmcol. Res.* 152:104609.

14. Zimmermann, J., Buchdunger, E., Mett, H., et al. 1997. Potent and selective inhibitors of the ABL-kinase: Phenylaminopyrimidine (PAP) derivatives. *Bioorg. Med. Chem. Lett.* 7:187–192.

15. Barker, A. J., Gibson, K. H., Grundy, W., et al. 2001. Studies leading to the identification of ZD1839 (IRESSA): An orally active, selective epidermal growth factor receptor tyrosine kinase inhibitor targeted to the treatment of cancer. *Bioorg. Med. Chem. Lett.* 11(14):1911–1914.

16. (a) Mayence, A. and Vanden Eynde, J. J. 2019. Baricitinib: A 2018 novel FDA-approved small molecule inhibiting Janus kinases. *Pharmaceuticals* 12:137. (b) Kalil, A. C., Patterson, T., Mehta, A. K., et al. 2020. Baricitinib plus Remdesivir for hospitalized adults with Covid-19. *N. Engl. J. Med.* Dec 11; NEJMoa2031994. doi: 10.1056/NEJMoa2031994.

17. Poratti, M., and Marzaro, G. 2019. Third-generation CDK inhibitors: A review on the synthesis and binding modes of Palbociclib, Ribociclib, and Abemaciclib. *Eur. J. Med. Chem.* 172:1243–153.

18. Menichincheri, M., Ardini, E., Magnaghi, P., et al. 2016. Discovery of entrectinib: A new 3-aminoindazole as a potent anaplastic lymphoma kinase (ALK), c-ros oncogene 1 kinase (ROS1), and pan-tropomyosin receptor kinases (Pan-TRKs) inhibitor. *J. Med. Chem.* 59:3392–3408.

Index

Note: Page numbers in *italics* indicate a figure and page numbers in **bold** indicate a table on the corresponding page.